THE MODERN BOOK OF STRETCHING

STRENGTH AND FLEXIBILITY AT ANY AGE

THE MODERN BOOK OF STRETCHING
STRENGTH AND FLEXIBILITY AT ANY AGE

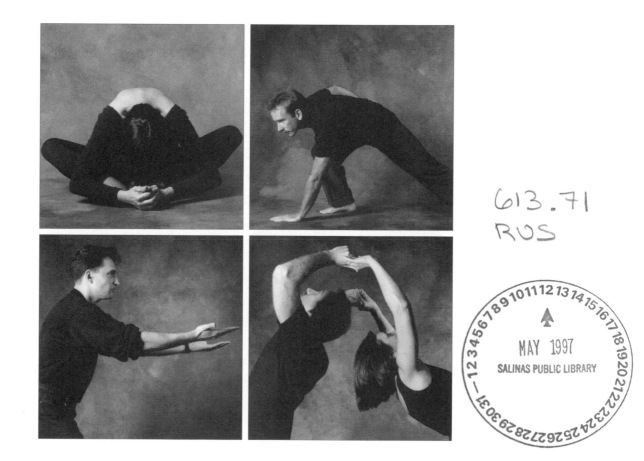

BY ANNE KENT RUSH • PHOTOGRAPHS BY PATRICK HARBRON

A BYRON PREISS BOOK

A DELL TRADE PAPERBACK

A BYRON PREISS BOOK

Published by Dell Publishing
a division of Bantam Doubleday Dell
Publishing Group, Inc.
1540 Broadway
New York, NY 10036

The Modern Book of Stretching: Strength and Flexibility at Any Age
by Anne Kent Rush; Photographs by Patrick Harbron
A Byron Preiss Book
0-440-50720-0

Book Design by Kenneth Lo

Printed in the United States of America
Published simultaneously in Canada
April 1997
10 9 8 7 6 5 4 3 2 1

PUBLISHER'S NOTE: This book contains certain exercises to aid
in the relaxation of the body. It does not make any specific medical
recommendations. Consult with a physician if you have any health questions.

*This book is
dedicated to
Sir Pelham Grenville Wodehouse
(1881—1975)
who truly understood flexibility.*

CONTENTS

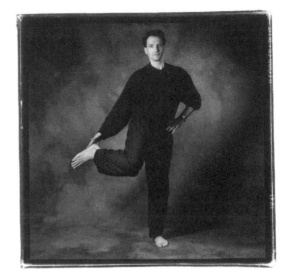

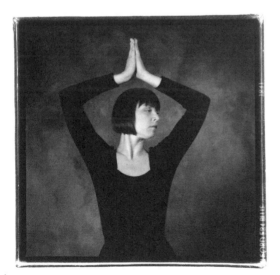

CONTENTS

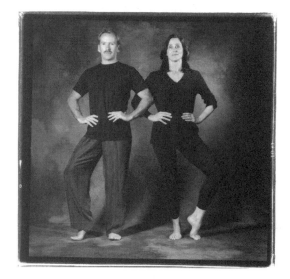

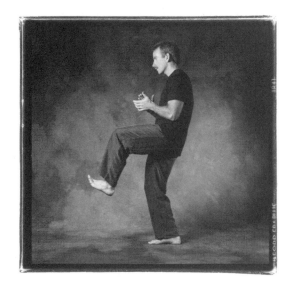

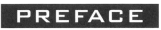

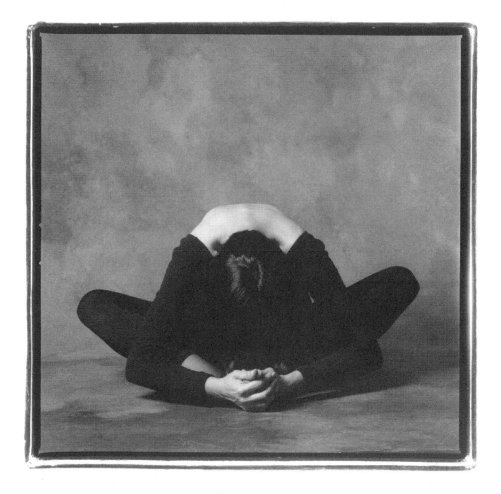

FUNDAMENTAL THINGS

PREFACE

FUNDAMENTAL THINGS

My dog wakes up slowly in the morning. He opens his eyes a bit to check if anyone has arisen. If the house is still and he needn't hurry, he uncurls from his sleeping position on the bed to stretch both paws in front of him. Next he straightens his back legs until he achieves a pose worthy of an Olympic gymnast. At the point of maximum extension, he arches his neck, angles his head and shoulders to one side, and rolls over. The grand finale to this wake-up ballet is to lie serenely on his back with all four paws in the air. This is a fine stretch. Clearly much pleasure is taken in the process.

When did we humans lose touch with our innate ability to wake up our muscles well and with feeling? If you pattern your pre-exercise stretching after a cat's or dog's (or jaguar's or bear's), you've chosen the perfect model. Animals know how to stretch smoothly and to the peak of their capabilities, not past, so that no tissue burns, tears, pulls, or cramps. Since we are also animals, the memory of how to move naturally through a stretch waits in our collective unconscious. Proper movement feels great, and we recognize it when we feel it. Ancient pleasures are recaptured. New horizons of physical action and mental calm open.

The exercises in this book come from my twenty-five years of researching and writing about preventive health care, and from the numerous training programs on psychology and exercise that I've taken and taught, from Aikido to Zen. The sequences in this book move from slow and easy to faster and more demanding as you progress. They are structured as dance patterns to make them more enjoyable as well as easier to remember and are accompanied by some of my favorite song lines. The stretches are designed to stimulate all the muscles and joints in your body. The way in which you move is the key to how fully your mind and body benefit—and to how much fun you have as you go. Enjoy.

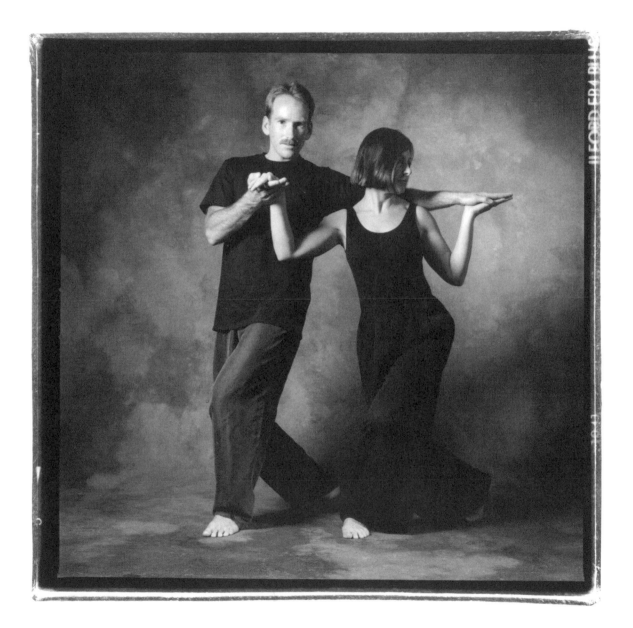

SLOW MOTIONS

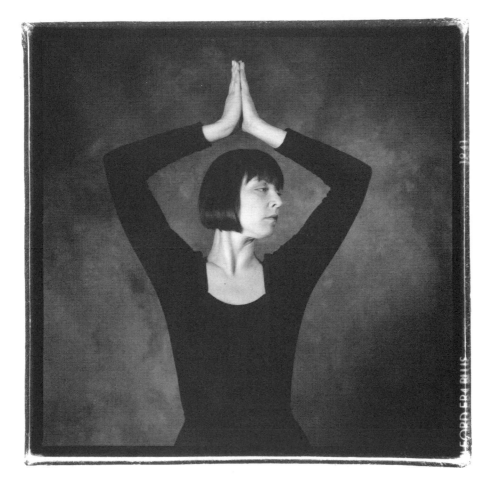

USE IT OR FUSE IT
A PROPER STRETCH
SLOW MOTIONS
BREATHE EASY
BACK BUILDERS

1

SLOW MOTIONS

USE IT OR FUSE IT

When you walk down the street with a happy-go-lucky beat...
What a wonderful way to start the day.
—Dietz & Schwartz

Grace and fluid motion are often assumed to be gifts to the young, but they are also rewards to the gracefully persistent. You can move comfortably at any age if you move well each day. Physical flexibility requires proper movement of every joint in your body, at least five days a week.

Why should we bother with this task? Because if we do not move an area, a host of problems can occur. Circulation gradually slows; waste materials build up rather than pass through; tendons and ligaments tighten and become brittle; skin loses its elasticity; muscle tone diminishes. Ultimately the joint can stiffen to the point of losing its ability to bend. Range of motion lessens, movements become jerkier, and comfort and pleasure in our body's locomotion wanes. If discomfort grows to pain, we may quit exercising altogether.

Time to start stretching. Better yet, begin before you hurt in order to prevent such miseries. Anyone at any age can increase mobility. You simply need to follow the guidelines in the Proper Stretch list that follows, and stay within your comfort zone to prevent strain.

Sleepy Stretches

Gentle stretching can help put you to sleep or wake you up. You can use the Slow Motions as a warmup and cooldown for other sports if you do them at a snail's pace. You can do the full routine at a fast pace for a complete workout. Start at a water ballet pace and gradually speed up, always keeping your rhythm.

You can avoid a common mistake when working out by remembering that stretching is NOT the same as warming up. If you stretch before raising your body temperature, you are likely to injure yourself. Warm up first with slow, steady movements that increase your heart rate. Then you can stretch your muscles as you speed up and feel warm.

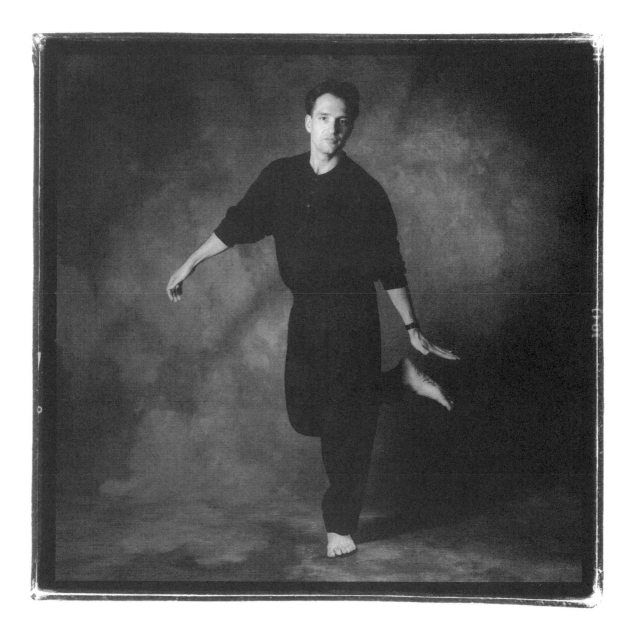

A PROPER STRETCH

Improper stretching is worse than no stretching at all and leads to injuries.
—Bob Anderson, ***Stretching***

Take these stretching guidelines to heart so you won't need to take your muscles to physical therapy:

DO NOT
- bounce; this tightens your muscles
- hold painful positions; this can tear your muscles
- exercise an injured area without consulting your physician
- favor one side or one direction of movement; this can lead to difficulties on the undeveloped side
- hold your breath; this starves your muscles of oxygen

DO, DO, DO
- move gently and smoothly; this builds strong muscles
- bend gradually and warm up to prevent strain
- control your action, rather than push or throw limbs
- pace yourself within your individual comfort zone

- monitor your tension areas so that while exercising one muscle, you do not unconsciously tighten another
- breathe with your motion; inhale as you stretch out; exhale as you bend in or release
- occasionally perform the routines at half a snail's pace to add an isometric element that builds strength
- sometimes perform the routine with speed to increase aerobic effect and coordination
- sprinkle single stretches throughout your day as relaxation breaks and stress management
- drink plenty of water
- experiment with stretching to music to keep your pace and to inspire you
- cool down

The fundamental things apply as time goes by.
—*Herman Hupfeld*

SLOW MOTIONS

Come and meet those dancing feet. . .
Hear the beat of dancing feet.
                    —Al Dubin

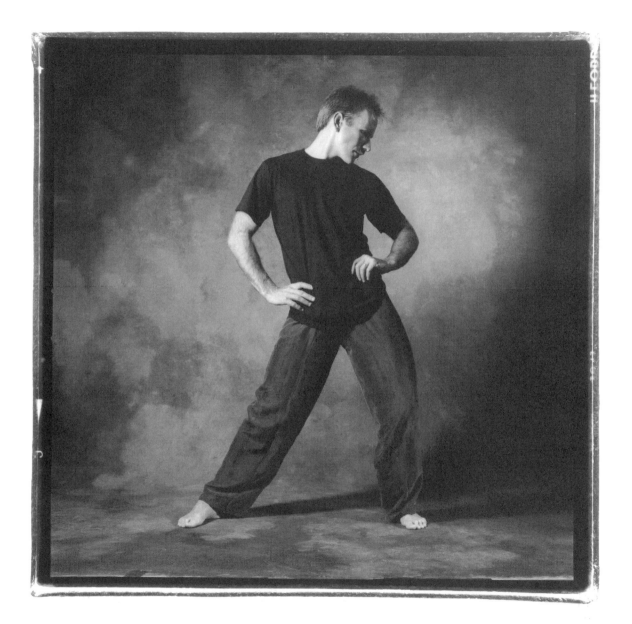

CLEOPATRA ROLL-LEFT

Erase royal neck pains.

This move relaxes the muscles of the neck, shoulders, and upper chest.

1. Stand with your feet about shoulder width apart. Look forward. Inhale as you raise both arms, palms up, from your sides. Straighten your spine, keeping your chest high and your lower back relaxed. Bring your palms together centered over your head.

2. Exhale as you turn your head left toward your left shoulder. Keep your elbows pressed back, in line with your shoulders.

3. Inhale as you roll your head back and allow your neck to relax so your head falls as far back onto your upper back as is comfortable. Exhale as you roll your head and neck toward the right shoulder.

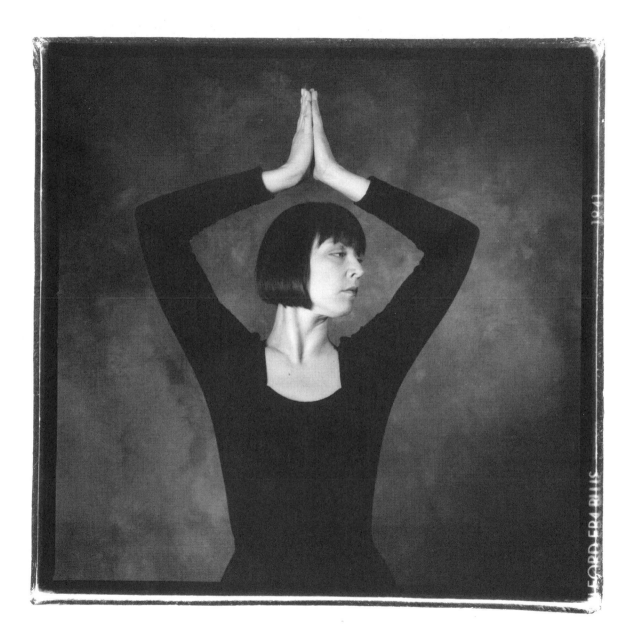

CLEOPATRA ROLL-RIGHT

Prevent mummy's neck.

4. Inhale as you raise your head up so that you are looking toward your right shoulder.

5. Exhale and bring your head facing forward. Try to keep your elbows pressed back and your body relaxed while you perform the head rolls.

6. To start another rotation, allow your head and neck to relax forward so you stretch the back of your neck in a new direction. Then roll your head to the left again. Perform three or four left head rolls.

7. Repeat this whole sequence moving your head in the opposite direction, circle right to left several times.

8. Roll very slowly to begin. Gradually speed up the pace only if you can comfortably maintain very smooth movement in your neck.

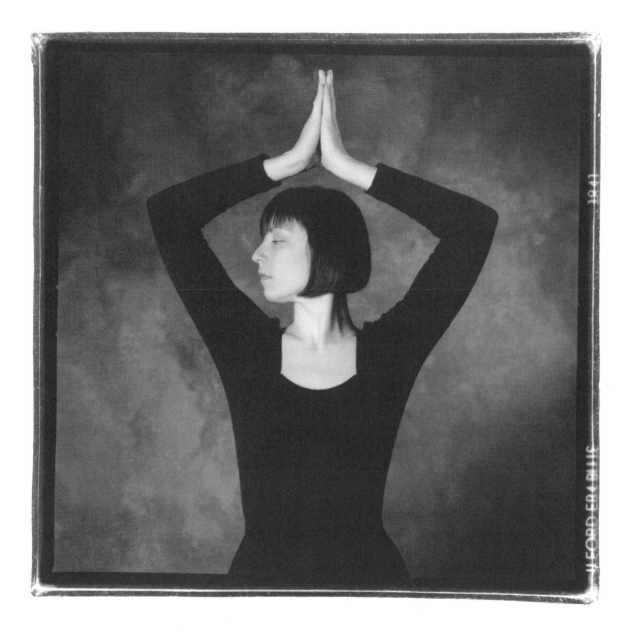

SHOULDER SNAKES

Stretch and slither.

This motion relaxes tight Trapezius muscles in the shoulders.

1. Bend your elbows close to your sides with upturned palms raised to a height just below your shoulders. Press both shoulders down slightly.

2. Keeping your head and neck upright, draw both shoulders backward.

3. Now raise both shoulders up toward your ears.

4. Allow your shoulders to relax forward and down. Repeat this cycle three or four times. Try to allow your movement to be smooth and continuous rather than jerky.

5. Do this movement in the opposite direction so that your shoulders roll, first, up and back, then, down and forward.

6. For more precise flexibility, you can snake each shoulder separately.

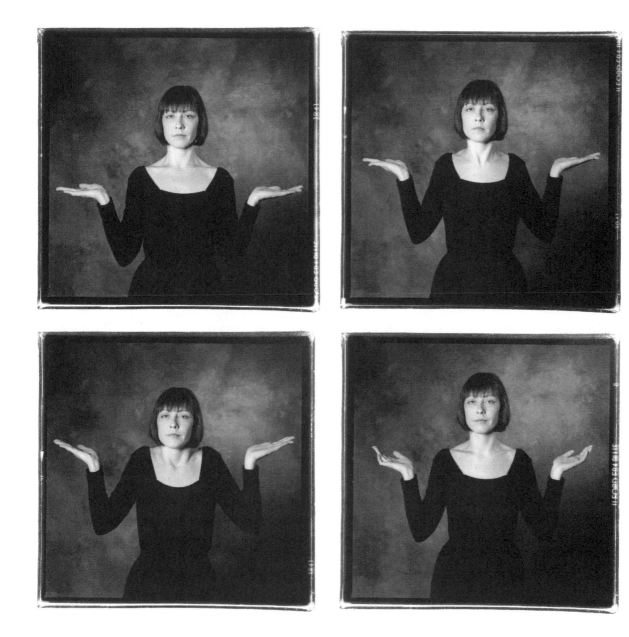

ELBOW HIP FLIP—RIGHT

Travolta movova.

This move stretches your waist and upper arms.

1. Stand with your feet together. Keep your bent elbows near your sides and make fists with both hands. Raise your hands to about shoulder height.

2. Now look to your right as you slide your right leg, toes pointed out, to the right. Tilt your torso to the right. Keep your elbows pressed outward at your sides and your fists beside your shoulders, not in front of you. Bring your right elbow as close to your right hip as is comfortable, and draw your left elbow as high up as possible.

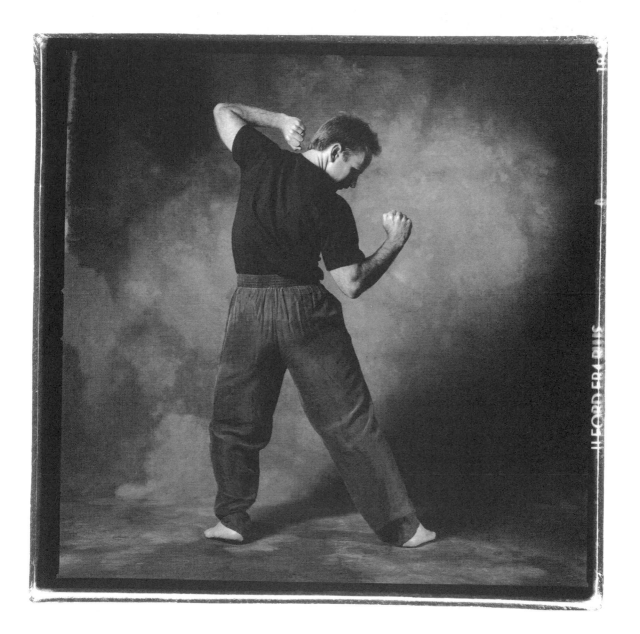

ELBOW HIP FLIP—LEFT

Day or night reliever.

3. To change directions, look forward again as you draw a half circle backward on the ground with your right toes, ending with your right foot next to your left foot as you began. To make this foot circle best, you'll need to lightly drag your toes along the ground, lifting your chest a bit. Press your buttocks out behind you as your leg moves back. Your pelvis tilts forward as your right foot slides forward beside the left foot.

4. Do the complete Elbow Hip Flip movement cycle to your left. Point your left leg to the left, as you draw your left elbow toward your left hip. Raise your right elbow above your right shoulder.

5. To change directions, press your hip backward as your left leg circles outward behind you with the toes sliding on the floor. Tilt your pelvis forward as you drag your left foot parallel to your right again.

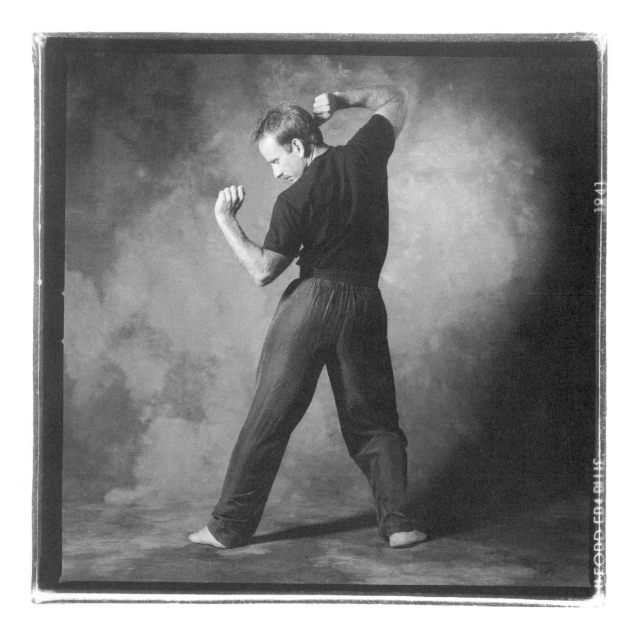

FOOT FANS

Your feet will love them.

This move keeps your ankles flexible.

1. Stand with your feet about a foot apart. Rest your weight on your left leg. Bend your knees slightly. Rotate the toes of your right foot outward.

2. Lift the right toes off the ground a bit as you rotate on your heel and fan your toes back toward the arch of your left foot. Repeat this back and forth fan motion several times.

3. Come to the center again with both feet. Shift your weight onto your right foot. Now do the Foot Fans to your left with your left foot.

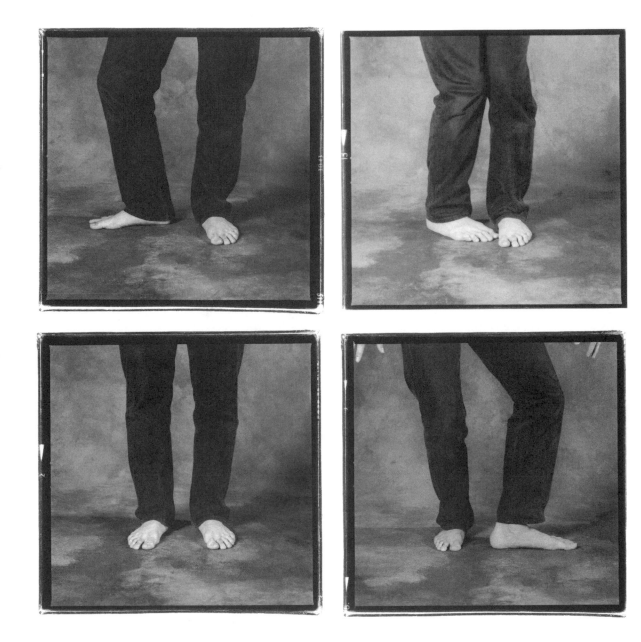

PIGEON

Double feet fans.

This move improves coordination.

1. Put your hands on your hips. Stand with your feet a bit more than a foot apart. Rotate on your heels as you turn the toes of both feet in toward each other. Bend your knees deeply as you do this keeping your right heel stationary and sliding your left foot to the left. This should move you a little to the left across the floor.

2. Now lean and shift your weight onto your left leg. Straighten your knees as you roll on your heels and flip the toes of both feet outward away from each other. Keep traveling in this left direction across the floor.

3. Now shift your weight onto the right leg and perform the Pigeon walk moving in the other direction across the floor. Try to keep your pelvis tucked under as you move.

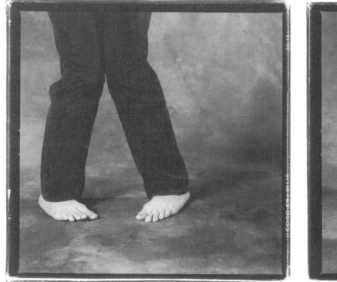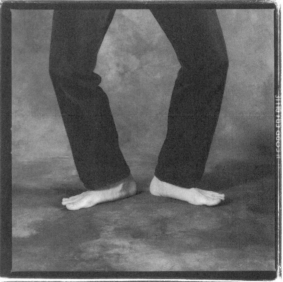

SIDE HOPS

▬▬

Both now.

This motion stretches your waist, hips, and arms.

1. Face forward, with your elbows bent and held near your waist. Keep heels of palms pressed out in front of you.

2. While keeping your hands, arms, head, and torso facing forward, jump up and turn both feet so that your hips turn to your right and your torso faces forward. This motion will cause you to twist at the waist.

3. With the torso and hands still facing forward, jump up again and swing your feet to your left. Land with toes pointing left. To help your balance, draw your arms in toward your torso as you jump up. Press your arms and hands forward and away from you as you land. Repeat these hops as often as they are fun and comfortable.

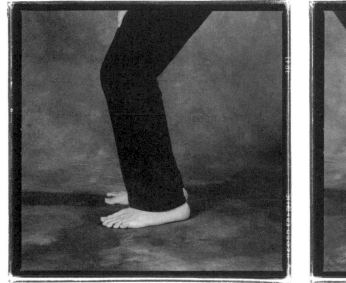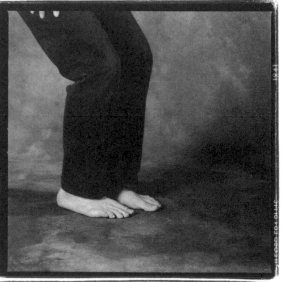

HEEL STOMPS

Flamenco finish.

This motion stretches your foot muscles and strengthens your legs.

1. Stand facing forward, knees bent and feet a few inches apart. Rest your weight on your right leg. Lift your left heel up while keeping your toes flat in place.

2. Now sharply press your left heel to the floor. At the same time, raise your right heel up and shift your weight onto your left foot.

3. Alternate these heel stomps several times as you bend your knees and hold your body straight above you. Experiment with different rhythms.

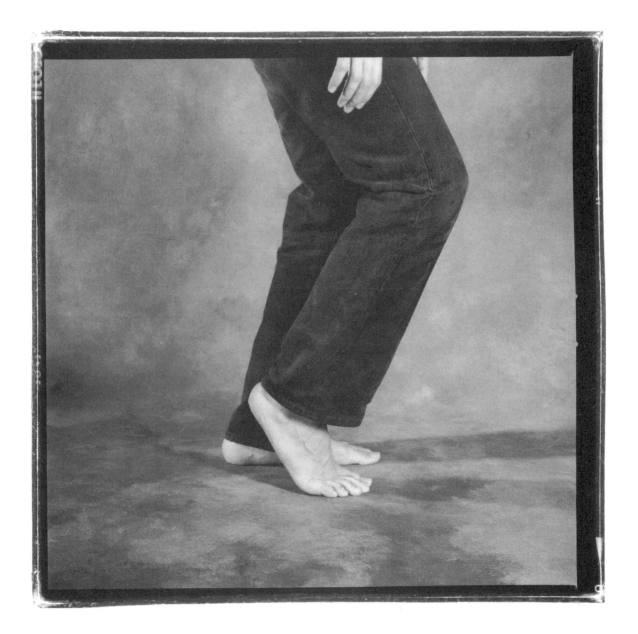

BREATHE EASY

Let yourself go; relax and let yourself go.
—Irving Berlin

The breath is at the core of body rhythm, and, like a snowflake, each person has a unique natural pattern. Rhythm is an aspect of a person's metabolism to which others often have strong reactions. You can like or dislike someone because he or she is speedy or slow paced, erratic or consistent. If you learn to recognize your own rhythm, you can broaden your insight into your moods, gain more control over your physical states, increase your ability to minimize stress, and improve your athletic performance.

Notice that when you are active you breathe relatively fast and high in your chest. Holding your breath is a sign of tense anticipation. Slow breathing is an aspect of relaxation and repose. Deep breathing is an aspect of deep emotion. Most of the time we let our breathing rhythms occur unconsciously, without being aware of how much they affect our moods.

If you reverse this process and change your breathing rhythm consciously from time to time, you'll find you can alter your emotional states considerably. Knowledge of breathing is a useful relaxation skill in any situation, without need for privacy, equipment, or extra time.

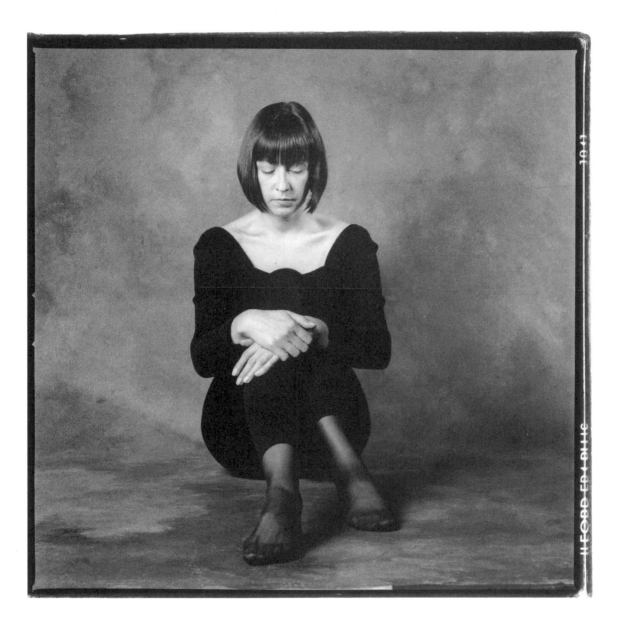

I Got Rhythm

The lungs need exercise to function well, just as joints and muscles do. Exercise demands more oxygen supply to our muscles, and deep breathing increases the flow.

The volume of our daily intake of air is five times greater than our daily intake of food and fluid. Because we need to clear the lungs of stale air to make space for fresh air, we need to be sure to exhale fully. In general, do not hold your breath during exertion. Inhale as you stretch out; exhale as you bend or pull in.

In general, you want to make very tiny movements of the sore body part. Synchronize the motions with your breathing. Inhale as you lift or stretch. Exhale as you release or bend. Most tension release occurs on the exhalation, as your muscles, "let go."

FINDING YOUR NATURAL BREATH RATE

You first need to learn to find the natural breathing rhythm you would have if no outside influences interfered. The Basic Breath exercise that follows teaches you how to do this. Once you have a sense of your own relaxed rhythm, you have a middle point from which to gauge variations in a spectrum from very tense to very relaxed. Any time you want to relax, it's simple to do the Basic Breath and improve your state.

The Basic Breath can be used for healing—to increase circulation in an area, to speed up tissue regeneration after injury, to relieve the pain of headaches and backaches, and to help you sleep. It also can be used to dramatically improve your physical agility and coordination by giving you sensitivity to and control over your body rhythms.

THE BASIC BREATH

The Basic Breath exercise was developed by Magdalene Proskauer, a San Francisco therapist. This breathing cycle is designed to trigger your natural rhythm gradually. By using this cycle you can let go of imposed rhythms and allow your own rhythm to surface. Find yourself while floating on air.

Lie on your back on the bed or floor. Relax your arms at your sides and let your feet fall out to the sides. Close your eyes and feel the way you are lying. Notice whether any part of your body feels a bit tense or doesn't seem to be resting comfortably on the surface beneath you. Now move your focus inside your body and notice where you feel movement as you breathe.

If you feel tense anywhere, try imagining that you can breathe into the tension, as though you could actually exhale through that body part. Imagine the breath relaxing your sore muscles as it moves through them. Breathing into a body part is something you can do anywhere, anytime you feel tense or nervous. Locate the tight place and "breathe into it." Breathe in sync with the tensing (inhale) and relaxing (exhale) of your movement.

As you are doing this exercise, loosen your clothing if it is tight at the waist. Let the muscles of your stomach and abdomen relax and let your breath sink lower in your body. Place one palm down at the lowest part on your torso where you can feel the motion of your breathing. Let your hand rest on this place until you begin to feel the rise and fall of your body under your palm from your breathing. Now let your hand and arm relax at your side again. If you see any pictures of yourself or other images during this breathing exercise, remember them and draw or write them down later. They are waking dreams and can be clues to your deeper feelings about yourself and your environment. You can interpret them as you would your other dreams.

Relax your jaw and open your mouth a little so that you can exhale through your mouth. You don't need to breathe heavily. Relax and breathe naturally. Inhale through your nose; exhale through your mouth; and pause at the end of the exhalation before you breathe again.

THE PAUSE

This pause is the key to the effectiveness of the breathing. Crucial things are happening to your body during the pause; you are actually still exhaling, though you may feel as though nothing is going on. Deepening your exhalation gets all the stale air out of your lungs and makes more room for fresh air when you inhale. Most of us don't exhale deeply enough. Often, when you feel that you can't take in enough air and that you'd like to inhale more deeply, it's because you haven't exhaled fully enough to make room in your lungs for new air. This is usually the breathing difficulty in asthma. Lengthening your exhalation can help release asthmatic symptoms.

You have paused at the end of the exhalation for a long time now. Let yourself really explore the pause. How does it feel to you? Does it feel too long? Not long enough? Are you a little worried that your body won't breathe in again unless you make it? Think of your breathing when you are asleep. You don't have to tell yourself to breathe then. Think of animals breathing when they are resting. Their breath is long and rolling. They don't tell themselves to breathe. You can learn to trust that your breath will always come in again.

Allow the pause to be as long as it wants. It may feel very long. See whether you can wait and stay with the pause until your body wants to breathe in again by itself. Inhale through your nose; exhale through your mouth; then pause and wait. It's a little like standing on the beach and waiting for another wave to come in. Try to find a pace at which you are neither holding your breath to prolong the pause nor making yourself breathe in again. Let yourself breathe in this pattern as long as you want.

This exercise in itself is deeply relaxing. If you have difficulty going to sleep, you can use this breath at night. Or anytime you feel tense you can take a few minutes off for yourself, relax, and find your rhythm again. The Basic Breath is a gentle, powerful centering exercise.

Every breath you take, every move you make . . .
—Sting

BACK BUILDERS

Treat me nice.
—Elvis Presley

Keeping the back flexible is one of the most important aims of any sound stretching program. Back pain usually results from imbalance of back muscle movement. Although the back bends naturally in four directions—forward, backward, sideways, and around—we tend to bend mainly forward. This lack of motion causes weakness and tension to develop in the other three muscle areas.

To head off back pains, use the vigorous stretching routines in this book plus the special back relaxers in this section. Pair your exercises so that you perform the opposite of each motion in sequence. When you do a forward bending exercise, follow it with a backward bending one. When you stretch to the right, next stretch to the left. If you hold the pose for some time, this adds an isometric element to build strength.

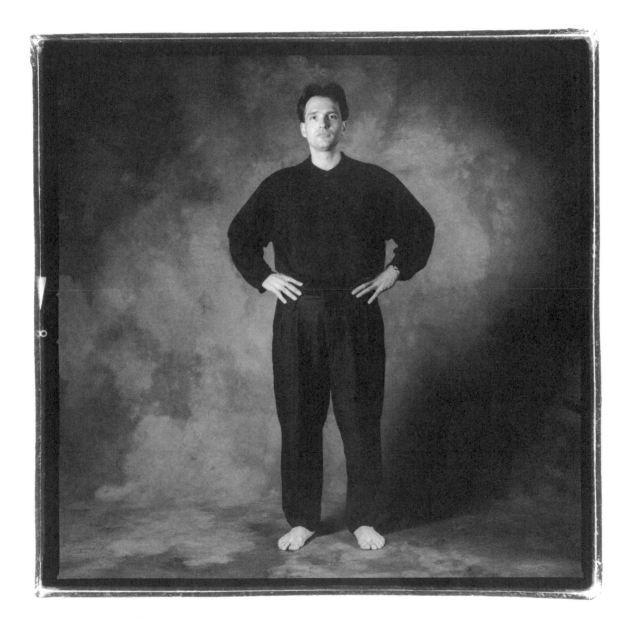

Back Care

Don't do any movement unless it feels completely comfortable, doesn't hurt or cause any strain. Work up slowly to difficult postures. In general, if you have any questions, consult your physician for a professional opinion.

Always warm up, cool down, and do lots of rests in between. Be careful. Specific exercises can provide extra stress on an injured body part. Don't do any exercise that applies pressure to the head if you have a neck problem, high blood pressure, back pain or injury, eye problems or are menstruating. Don't do severe back bends if pregnant. All these conditions apply inappropriate pressure.

Incorrect forward stretching can aggravate sciatica. Be sure to extend the spine upward and bend at the waist before you stretch forward. Be careful you don't strain your knees by squatting too low or standing too long. If you recently had any illness or surgery, check with your physician before undertaking any exercise.

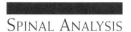

Spinal Analysis

Psychological associations with body parts are rooted in the parts' functions. The back bears burdens and thus is associated with a person's sense of limits and capacities for work or stress. A "backache personality" is often recognizable as overambitious or strongly prone to placing mind over matter. "Spineless," "no backbone," and "backing out" are phrases used about people we feel have shirked their rightful burdens.

Aim for a "back-rub personality" rather than a "backache personality." If you think you have a back problem that is caused largely by stress rather than physical trauma, it is still a priority to treat the physical symptom first. Often, after the physical symptom of a back problem is taken care of, the psychological problem surfaces. You can't ignore your body and function well. The body is one of your natural limits. If you respect a limit, it becomes a resource. Treat yourself to frequent back rubs and daily stretches. Back to basics.

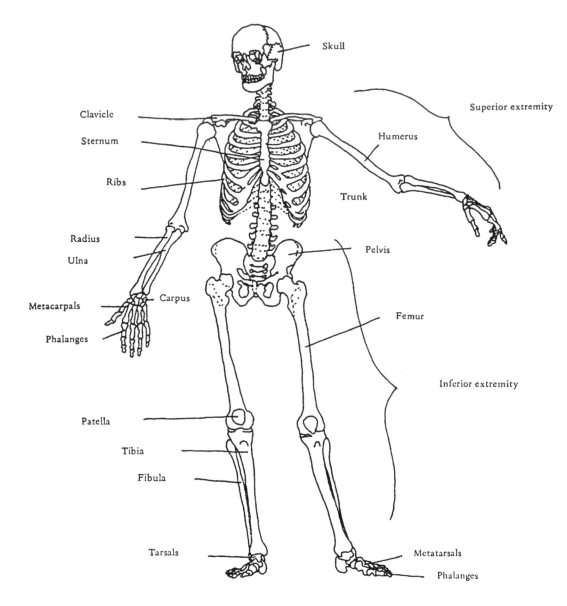

Skull

Superior extremity

Clavicle

Sternum

Humerus

Ribs

Trunk

Radius

Ulna

Pelvis

Metacarpals

Carpus

Femur

Phalanges

Inferior extremity

Patella

Tibia

Fibula

Tarsals

Metatarsals

Phalanges

SKELETON, FRONT VIEW

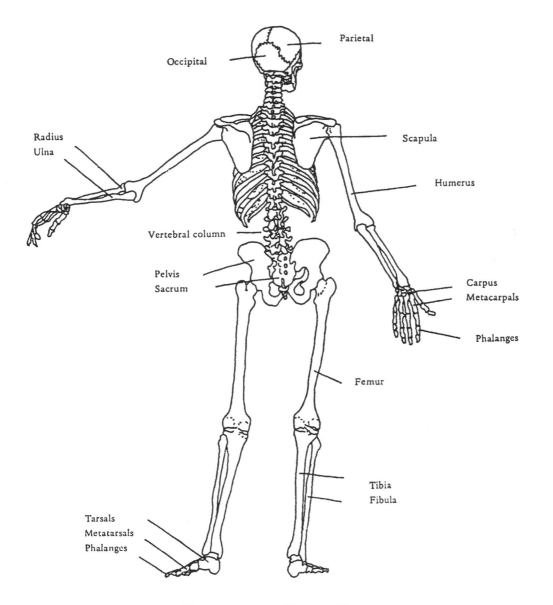

Occipital

Parietal

Radius
Ulna

Scapula

Humerus

Vertebral column

Pelvis
Sacrum

Carpus
Metacarpals

Phalanges

Femur

Tibia
Fibula

Tarsals
Metatarsals
Phalanges

SKELETON, BACK VIEW

NECK RELEASE

Curve ball.

This exercise is one of the most relaxing treatments for a tired or sore neck. It enables the neck and jaw muscles to relax and allows the neck vertebrae to realign.

1. Lie down on a pad on your back with your knees elevated by a pillow. Place a six-inch air-filled rubber ball under your neck. Find a place for the ball that allows you to give over the work of holding up your head completely to the ball.

2. The more you allow the ball rather than your neck muscles to support your head, the more aligned the vertebrae in your neck will become. Imagine that each time you exhale, you can send your breath into your neck muscles to relax them from the inside.

3. You can also roll your head slightly from side to side over the ball as you inhale and exhale to massage your neck muscles.

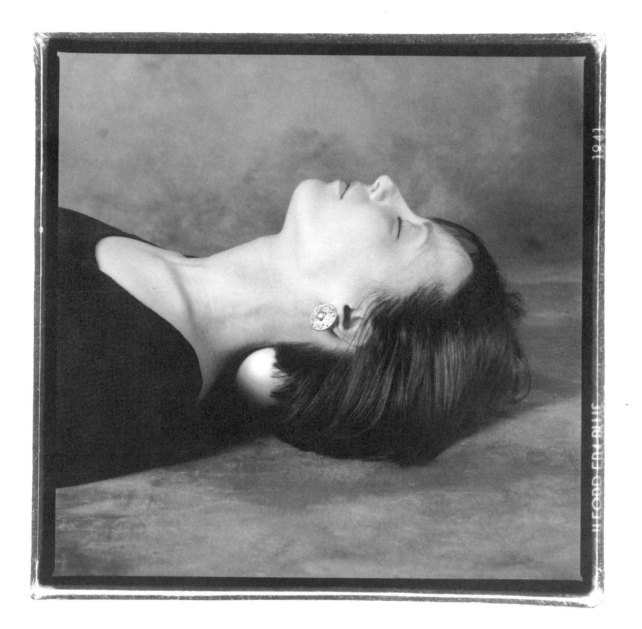

FULL SPINE RELEASE

◼︎◼︎

Head to tail.

A six-inch ball filled with air can give a great massage to different parts of your back. The angle of lift and the flexibility of the ball allows your lower back muscles to release tension. Lying on two balls at once allows your spine to stretch out and become suspended between the balls like a hanging bridge. As the space between the vertebrae increases, the spine lengthens and moves into alignment.

1. Place the ball under your neck as you did in the Neck Release.

2. Place a second ball under the base of your spine. Move the ball around until you find a place where your back feels completely comfortable when you put your weight on it. You can keep your feet on the floor. Or you can raise your knees to balance over your chest.

3. As you exhale, imagine that you can breathe down through the center of your spine and into the ball. With each breath, let your muscles relax more.

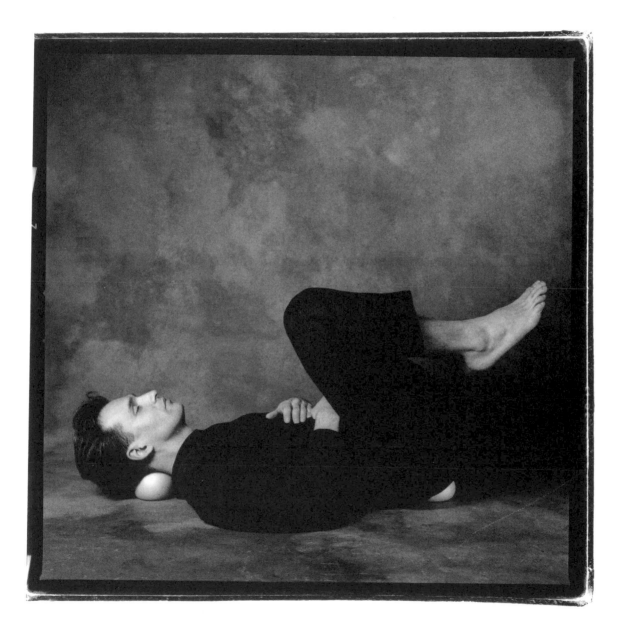

FROG FLEX

Then grip it.

This motion relaxes your hip joints and stretches thigh muscles.

1. Sit on a pad on the floor. Bend your knees and place the soles of your feet together. Clasp your toes with your palms.

2. Exhale as you lightly press your knees out and down toward the floor. Inhale as you draw them up again. Do not press your joints beyond a comfortable stretch, or bounce your legs, as this may cause muscle strain.

3. Start slowly and move rapidly as you feel comfortable. Maintain a smooth, continuous motion.

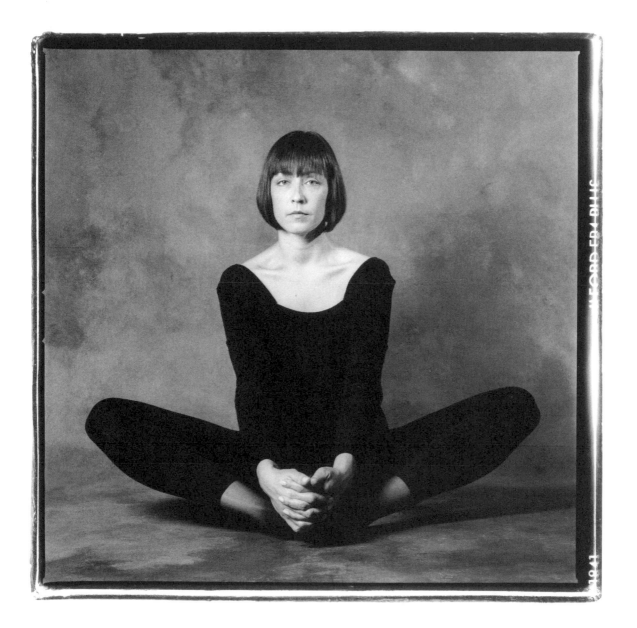

EGG BALL

Hatch a straight spine.

This exercise releases lower back tension and aligns your spine.

1. Sit on the floor with your knees bent and your ankles crossed comfortably in front of you. Place an air-filled rubber ball about six inches in diameter beside you. Relax your arms at your sides and place your hands in your lap. Close your eyes and make a mental note of where you feel the sitting bones of your pelvis resting against the floor. Allow your breathing to relax.

2. Lean forward. Raise your hips off the floor a bit and place the ball behind you under your hips. Rest your arms in your lap.

3. Lean back so you are sitting straight with your weight on the ball. Keep your eyes closed and focus on releasing your spine, back, and hip muscles. If the ball is in the right spot, you will feel no discomfort, and you will feel as though you can sit straight effortlessly. Move the ball until you find a comfortable position for you. Rest there awhile.

4. Notice where your hips and tailbone are pressing on the floor now. How has your sitting changed?

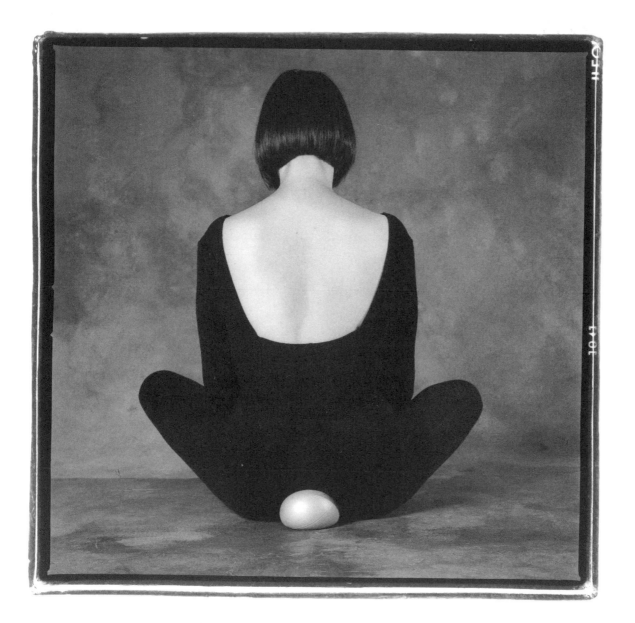

SQUAT REST

Sciatic sedative.

This position opens hip joints to release pressure on the lower back. It relieves pinching of the sciatic nerves, which lead from the base of the spine across the hips and down the legs.

1. With feet shoulder width apart, bend your knees and squat. Try to keep your heels flat on the floor and your feet parallel rather than turned out, or rest on your toes if this is more comfortable.

2. Fold your arms and rest your elbows on your knees. Relax in this position so that gradually your weight shifts more onto your shoulders and legs, and your back feels relaxed. If this position is easy, try the following more advanced squat position.

3. Press your elbows outward on the insides of your knees so your hip joints are stretched a bit. As you rest, your forehead can lean forward onto your clasped hands.

4. Gradually relax so that the position rather than muscle tension is holding you in place.

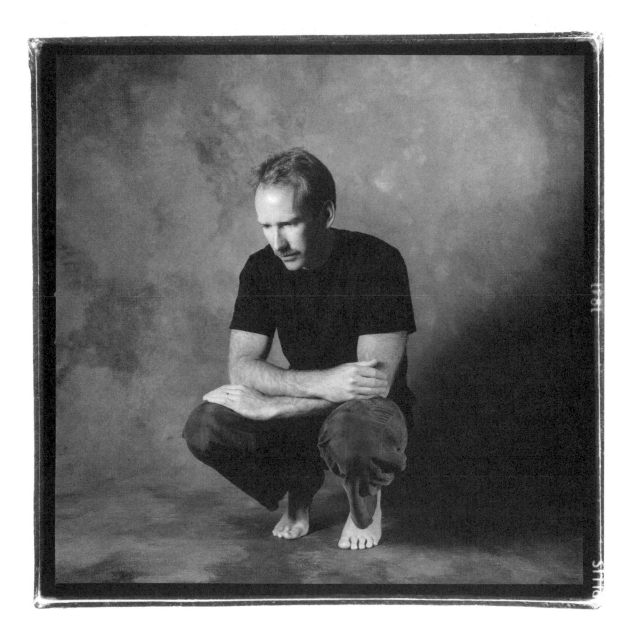

LILY

Fold your petals.

Now that your hip joints are loosened from the Frog Flex and the Squat Rest, try the Lily for a full back and leg stretch.

1. Sit on the floor with knees bent and the soles of the feet pressed together in front of you. Hold your toes in both palms.

2. Inhale as you straighten and then arch your back. Exhale as you lean forward over your legs. Bend more at the waist. Allow your head to relax toward your toes. Breathe quietly and slowly in this position. Unfold slowly.

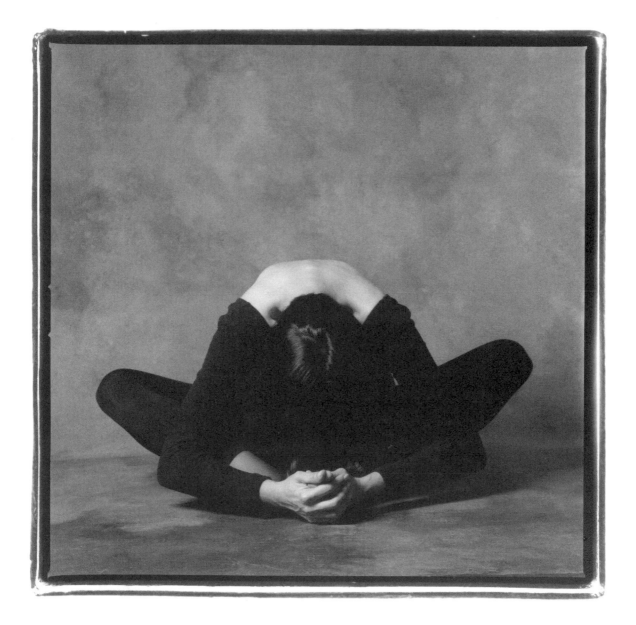

BACK REST

A flat-out favorite.

This rest can be done anytime for relaxation. It is good to lie down flat on your back following the Lily in order to release any muscle cramping from the forward stretch. You can simply lie down, or you can perform the full relaxation process. Practiced over time, this exercise will help you relax and sleep more deeply every night.

1. Lie down on your back on a flat floor pad or firm bed with your arms resting at your sides and your palms up.

2. Try to clear your mind of thoughts other than the feelings in your body. As you begin, make a mental note of how your body feels lying on the floor. You can compare this with your sensations at the end of the exercise. Notice which parts of your body are touching the floor and which parts seem held away. Do you feel tilted in any direction?

3. Starting with your feet, do a detailed observation of which body parts are resting fully on the ground and which are tightly

held up. Flex and release each joint separately and each muscle as you work your way up to the head. Inhale as you flex a muscle; exhale as you release.

4. Allow your breathing to massage you from the inside as though you could exhale down through your body and into any tight areas to soften them.

5. If you are still awake when you reach your neck and head, compare how your body feels resting on the floor to when you started.

SOLO PERFORMANCES

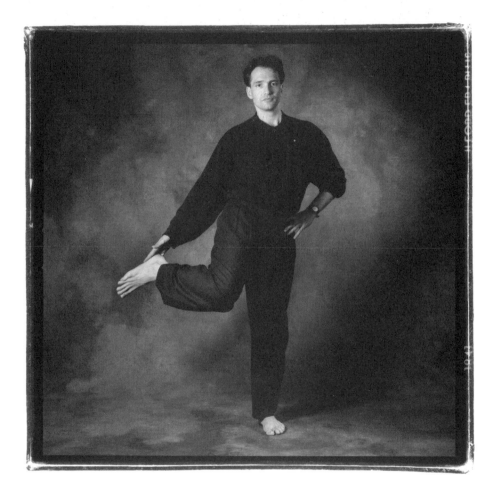

MIND MATTERS
VISUALIZATION
BREATHE FOR ACTION
WAKE-UP FLEXES

SOLO PERFORMANCES

MIND MATTERS

Something inside of me started a symphony…
All nature seemed to be in perfect harmony.
—James Hanley

The mind is like a muscle that enjoys stretching as much as other body parts do. The human head weighs between fourteen and eighteen pounds, giving your neck quite a job to hold it up all day. Exercises can strengthen the neck muscles and improve the blood flow to your brain. Good circulation to your head not only stimulates your gray matter, it also improves the functioning of your whole body because the brain controls and orders your muscle activity. The brain is the boss.

VISUALIZATION

Visualization in the realm of exercise refers to using healthy, flexible images of your body to improve your physical condition and performance. Through this process, your mind can revive your flagging muscle power and help smooth tight muscles.

There are two steps in the process. If you have a torn ligament, allow yourself to see an image in your mind's eye of the current state of that body part, imagining what the area looks like fragmented and inflamed. Next visualize how it should be. Looking at anatomy charts is useful. Throughout the day bring this healthy picture of your ligaments and muscles to mind to encourage healing.

This mental process of visualization is an ancient technique, which shamans, yogis, witches, and other healers have used well throughout history. Many Western medical doctors now use visualization effectively to help cancer patients and injured athletes. Visualization is useful for people who are in pain, too tired, or too sick to do other kinds of treatments or exercise. You can also try encouraging healing in other people by visualizing them healthy.

Visualization can be used as a form of practice that will improve your performance. Athletes often use visualization as part of their warmup routines. Visualize yourself doing an exercise or sport before the event. Imagining something stimulates many of the same responses in your nerves and muscles as doing it. You can also use visualization throughout the day as a preventive technique by maintaining a healthy image of your body in top shape.

MIND MASSAGE

Visualization can be used to explore an emotional or physical pain or tight muscle. Imagine you can shrink yourself and walk into your body to search and do internal maintenance. Don't preplan the story; simply try to let the events occur. They will.

Lie down, close your eyes, and relax your breathing. If you have a specific ache or pain you want to work on, locate it and then choose a natural body opening as your "entranceway." Imagine you can shrink yourself or someone else to about a half inch or smaller.

The journey in and out is just as important as the destination. Resist hurrying or missing any steps. You can talk out loud about what you are doing and how it feels to you. If you have a pain in your upper back you want to reach, you could enter through your mouth. Look around at the setting and describe it. "I am walking up to the mouth. I am crawling over the lips. As I let myself down inside, the surface becomes slippery. It's dark in here. I'm walking toward the back of the mouth on the teeth. They feel sharp and bumpy."

When you reach the back of the mouth, decide how to get down the throat and into the shoulder. "There's a deep hole here like a well. There's no way to get down except jump, but I don't know where I'll land." You can decide to go on or try another way. "I think I'll just jump." Describe your descent, what you see, how you feel. Almost always a surprise landing takes place; if not, pick something to catch onto to stop yourself when you feel you've fallen far enough.

When you land, decide how you're going to get to your sore muscle. You can swim through an artery or walk along a tendon. When you reach the sore muscle, look around. Describe what you see. Try to imagine a way you could massage the muscle by walking on it or squeezing it. Imagine you are doing this. Take your time.

When you have massaged to your satisfaction, begin your journey out of the body. Out again, imagine you can expand to your normal size and merge with your larger body. Take a moment to check how the previously sore muscle feels now. Often it feels greatly relaxed.

In the night when I feel blue . . .
All I have to do is dream,
Dream, dream, dream, dream . . .
—Boudleaux and Felice Bryant

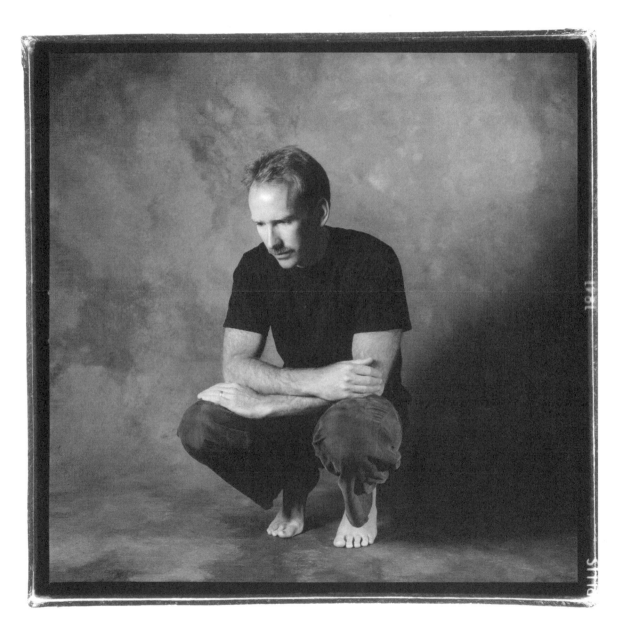

Stress Management

It lifts you up when you're run down.
—Vernon Duke

The conclusion of a study on stress conducted by Richard Lazarus and his colleagues at the University of California (UC), Berkeley, is that relatively minor yet frequent annoyances have a more destructive effect on our health than do grand-scale traumas. With stress, it's the little things that mean a lot.

The good news is that small tension-relief sessions performed frequently throughout the day can have a big effect on relieving stress. Make healing a way of life. Include short stretching and breathing breaks in each day's routine to keep the little stresses from snowballing. Take a moment to bend over in your chair and relax your back several times a day. Sprinkle brief exercises throughout your daily routine. You'll be doing yourself a big preventive favor.

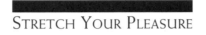

Stretch Your Pleasure

Another UC (Berkeley) study found that to be free of stress it's not enough to eliminate negative factors from your life. You have to *add* positive ones. This is a program worth lots of attention.

Fill your life with treats, luxuries, and happy experiences. Lavish your loved ones with small signs of affection and big treats. Up your pleasure quota. Remember, exercise is to stress as a bath is to a day's dirt. Keep your body feeling great. Get used to being good to others and to yourself. Doctor's orders.

> *It's been a hard day's night*
> *I've been working like a dog. ...*
> *But then I come home to you.*
> *You know the things that you do*
> *Make me feel alright.*
>   *—John Lennon and Paul McCartney*

BREATHE FOR ACTION

Now that you know the Basic Breath (page 32), you can apply it to all your stretching exercises and even to pain relief. As you imagine you are breathing into a body part, you stimulate circulation in that area. More blood flows to the painful spot, warming it, bringing more oxygen to decrease aching, carrying away waste materials from the cells, and generally reviving and relaxing the tissue. What you usually sense as a result of breathing into the body part is a warming and softening of the muscle and sometimes a tingling sensation from the change in circulation. This relaxation of the tissue will immediately cause some relief of your aches and pains. For relief of severe pain, continue the breathing process longer. No body part is unreachable by the breath.

Adding a small movement to your breathing exercise can also increase its effectiveness at relieving pain. Although you need not be in any particular position, the quickest pain relief comes from doing the exercise while lying down, because you can give over the work of holding up your weight to the bed or floor and put all your attention on relaxing.

Synchronize the motions with your breathing. Inhale as you lift or stretch. Exhale as you release or bend. Most tension release occurs on the exhalation, as your muscles "let go."

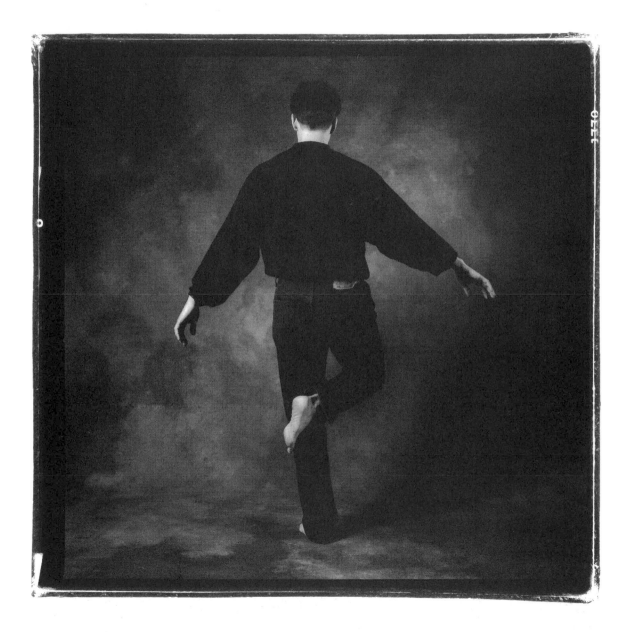

PALM SPHERE

Current circles.

We have modern scientific equipment that can locate and measure electro-magnetic currents in the body. Centuries ago martial arts masters, healers and yogis felt these subtle currents during their practice and included systems for directing the currents to deepen the energizing effects of their movements. You can do a simple exercise with your hands to feel these currents. The experience offers you a way to heighten the scope and extend the range of your movements and send energy all over your body. Initially try this technique with your hands. Later you can try directing the energy to any part of your (or someone else's) body.

1. Sit comfortably, eyes closed, hands resting palms up on your knees. Relax any tense muscles you feel by imagining that each time you exhale, a little more tension leaves your body. Allow your breathing to sink low in your body so that your belly puffs out a bit as you inhale and sinks back in as you exhale.

2. Now imagine what it would feel like if you could send your exhalation through the center of your body, through your torso, to massage your muscles from the inside. Allow your breath to bring warmth and air to any tight areas. As you breathe, oxygen is drawn into your body and spreads to various parts through your bloodstream.

3. As you exhale, imagine you can send air down through your shoulders and arms and eventually into your hands. What would it feel like if you could exhale down your arms and out the center of your palms, through a spot about the size of a quarter?

4. Raise your palms so they are facing each other at about waist height. The increased circulation to your hands as a result of your breathing sometimes brings a sense of warmth and tingling. The muscle relaxation and improved circulation allow the body's electric currents to move more easily. Can you feel any sense of this electric flow between your facing palms?

5. Some positions intensify the current flow. Allow your hands to move slowly in any direction they want. Try holding them different distances apart to see where the current feels stronger and where it weakens. You may sense a flexible shape to the air space. Sometimes it feels as though you are holding a ball between your hands.

6. The more you relax and direct your breathing down your arms, the stronger the sensation will become. You will notice that this process releases tension in your shoulders and arms.

7. You can use this directed breathing to relax tight muscles in other parts of your body as you move. Being able to send this energy to different parts of your anatomy gives you a resource for reviving tired muscles and spirits.

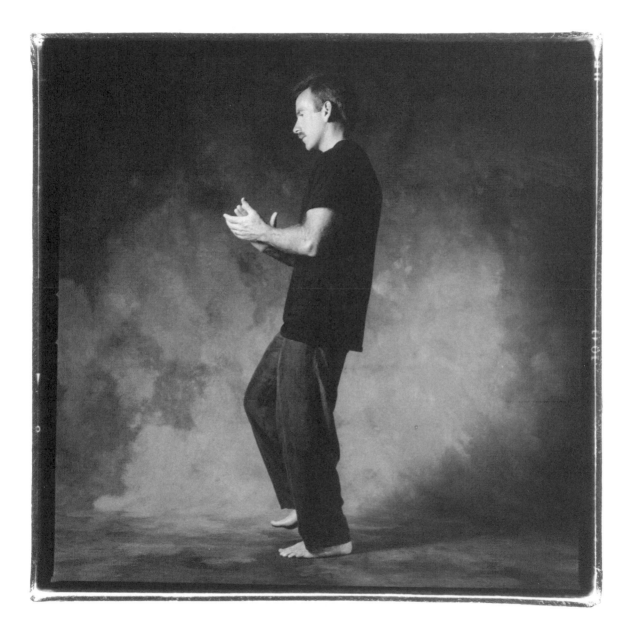

WAKE-UP FLEXES

Oh, how I hate to get up in the morning.
—Irving Berlin

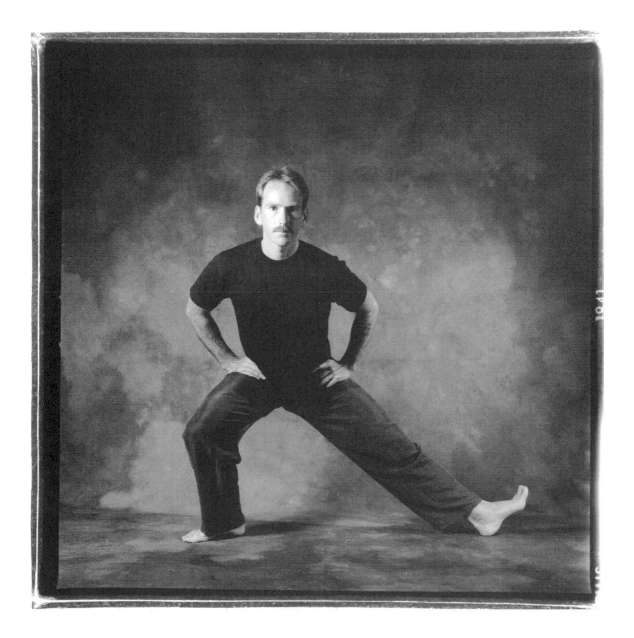

LEG ROCK

Everybody let's. . . .

This movement relaxes arm, leg, and knee joints.

1. Stand with your legs a bit more than shoulder width apart. Face forward and keep your torso upright. Bend your right knee and lean to your right side. Stretch out your right arm about chest height to your right side.

2. Lean back to center over your two feet and clap.

3. Bend your left knee and lean to your left. Stretch out your left arm in that direction.

4. Come back to center and clap.

5. Stretch out your right arm to the side as you lean to your right and bend your right knee. Keep alternating sides about eight times to loosen your arm and leg muscles for the Leg Leans that follow.

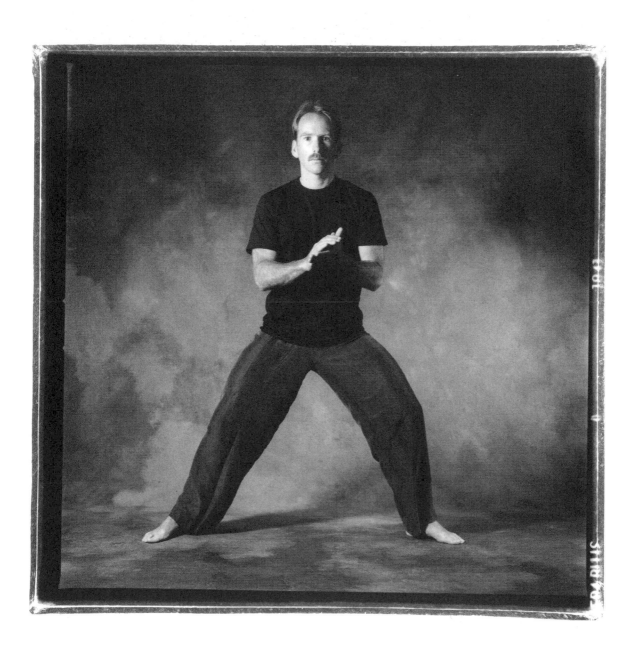

LEG LEAN—LEFT

It's a long way to tip of bare toes.

This movement focuses on stretching inner thigh muscles and the Achilles tendon in your heel. Protect your knees from strain by being careful not to extend your knee beyond your foot unless you have been training for quite awhile.

1. Place your hands on your hips. Face forward and inhale. Shift your weight onto your right leg, exhale, and bend the right knee. Stretch your left leg out to your left. Flex the left toes up, and bend the right knee more to accentuate the leg muscle stretch. Try to keep your torso upright; resist the impulse to lean forward.

2. Inhale as you roll your weight onto your left foot. Lean your body a bit to your left to bring your weight centered on both feet again. You should be standing in the center as you began with neither leg stretched to the side.

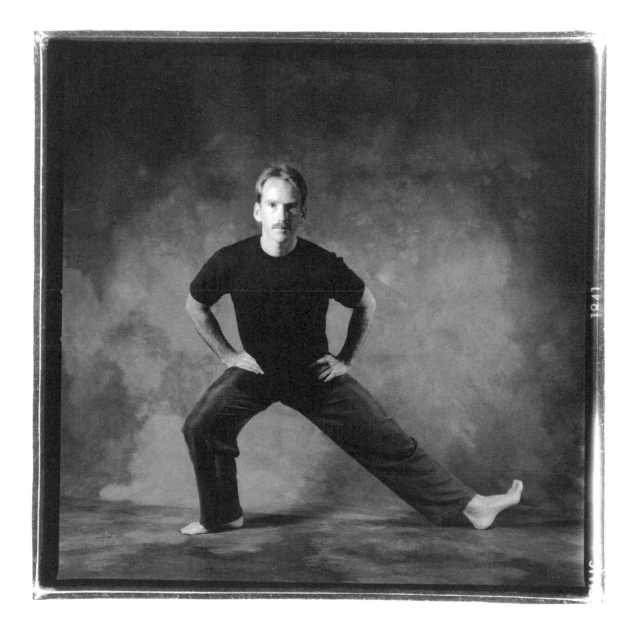

LEG LEAN–RIGHT

It's a long way by bone.

1. Now lean further to your left as you bend that knee and exhale.

2. Stretch your right leg out to your right. Flex the toes up.

3. Inhale as you return to your center stance.

4. Now begin the whole sequence again to your right, but this time do not stop in the center between leans. Alternate right and left, making one smooth, continuous motion.

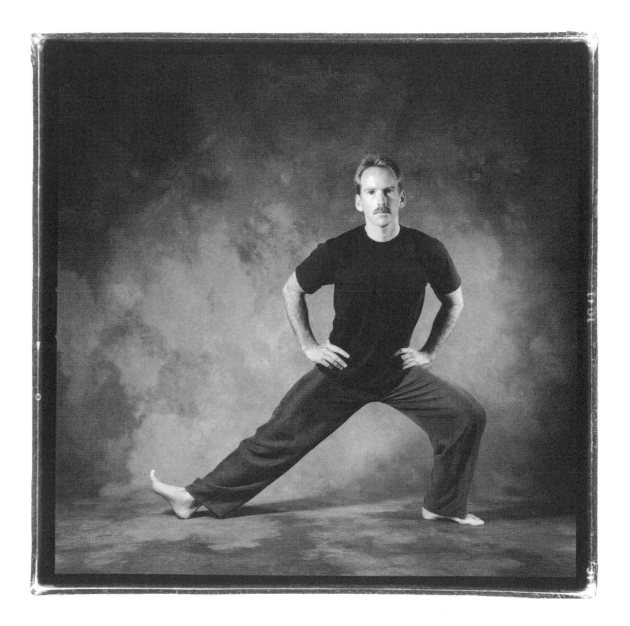

BODY PULL

■■■■■

Funny hop.

This movement stretches arm and torso muscles.

1. Stand firmly with your feet about shoulder width apart and your knees slightly bent. Lean forward at the waist as you stretch both arms in front of you with palms up at chest height.

2. Quickly flip your palms over toward the floor and make fists as you pull your elbows back toward your body. As you pull your arms back, hop forward a bit on the floor. End with your elbows snug to your waist and your fists clenched.

3. Repeat so that you move forward across the floor with these hops. Really stretch your arm muscles as you reach and pull.

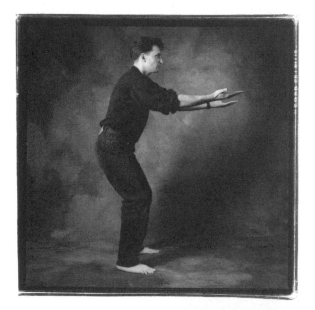

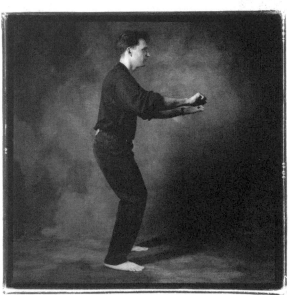

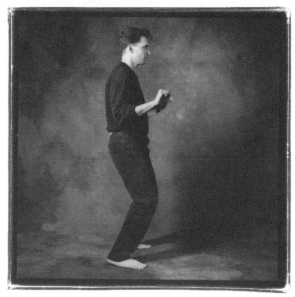

HIP SLAP

████████

Tush push.

This is a good stretch for your shoulders, back, and waist.

1. Place your feet about shoulder width apart. Try to keep your hips facing forward as you turn your torso. In one continuous movement, look to the left and behind you as you swing your left arm around. Slap your right hip with your left palm. Keep this palm in place.

2. Next swing your right arm in front of you and slap your left hip with your right palm.

3. Look to your right and perform the Hip Slap as you swing to your right.

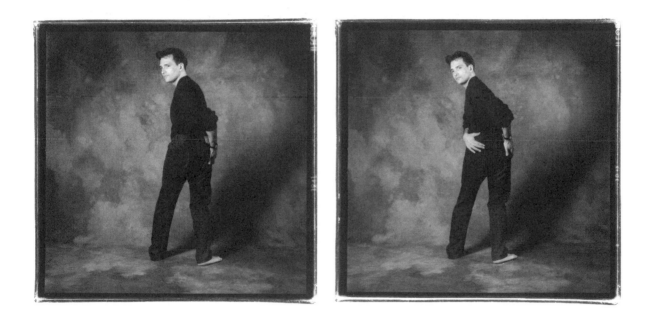

HEEL ROCK

Then roll.

This movement strengthens your foot and ankle muscles and stretches your calves.

1. With your feet only a few inches apart, rock forward on both feet so your weight is on your toes and your heels are off the ground. Lift high enough to feel your calf muscles grip. Balance with your arms out to your sides or on your hips.

2. Lean back and roll your weight onto your heels so your toes are off the ground. Flex your toes up enough so you can feel your calf muscles stretch.

3. Alternate forward and backward rolls.

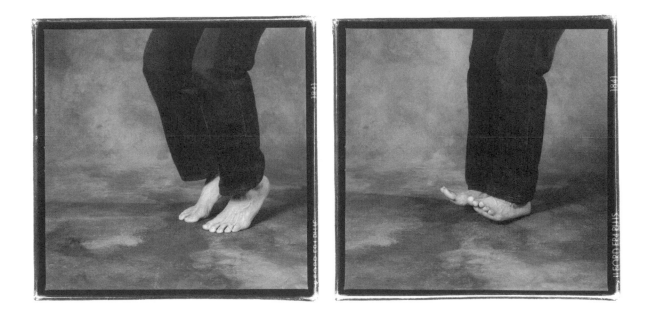

SOLE SLAP

Easier in a kilt.

This stretch helps keep your knees limber and improves coordination.

1. Stand with your weight on your left leg and your arms out to your sides or on your hip. Bend your right knee and flip your right foot up behind your left leg. Slap the sole of your right foot with your left palm.

2. Touch down again with your right foot. Balancing on your left leg, turn your right knee in as you bend it and flip your right foot out to the right. Slap the sole of your right foot with your right palm.

3. Touch down again with your right foot. Then bend the knee and flip the right leg in front of your left leg. Slap the sole of your right foot with your left palm. Repeat the whole sequence with the opposite leg.

4. For more of a challenge, switch direction and leg each time you sole slap. You will change your standing leg with each new Sole Slap. Done quickly, the step resembles a Scottish dance.

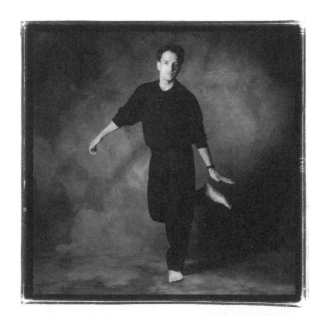

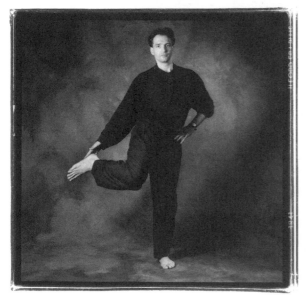

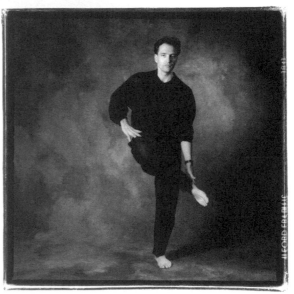

STEP SLIDE HOP

Hard to stop.

This exercise relaxes your arms and legs.

1. Step down on your right foot as you lift your left off the floor.

2. Slide the sole of your left foot forward across the floor as you shift your weight onto the left foot and move forward.

3. Then raise your right foot off the floor as you hop in place with your left.

4. Stomp in place once with your right foot and clap. Then stomp once with your left and clap. Repeat this sequence several times.

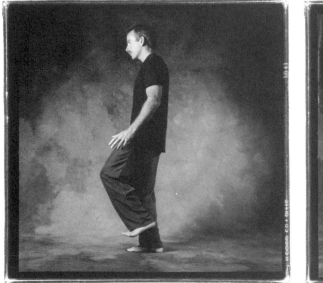

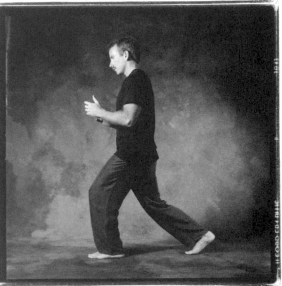

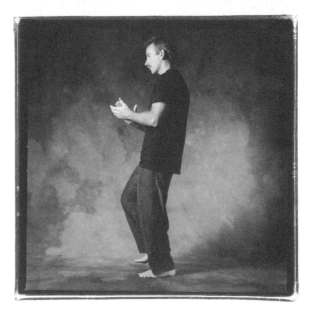

GRAND FINALES

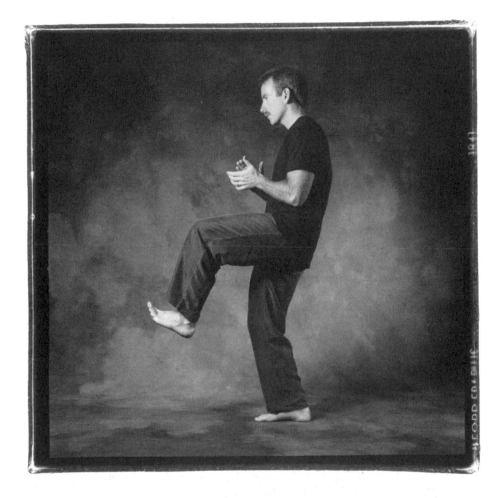

THE MUSCLE AND BONES OF IT
ENERGY STRETCHING
ENERGY CENTERS
HIGH STRETCHING

GRAND FINALES

THE MUSCLES AND BONES OF IT

To know how to dance is to know how to control oneself.
—Fred Astaire to Ginger Rogers in Swing Time

After you've been performing the stretches awhile, you may want to know more about which parts of your body you are actually moving. The human skeleton has 206 bones, which need exercise to maintain their mass. Without weight-bearing exercise, bones start to lose their density and become thinner and more fragile. Ligaments hold the bones together and are covered with cartilage. The body has 600 different muscles, often paired in extenders and flexors. All these aspects of the body need exercise to function well.

Pain offers no gain, because if the muscles are overworked or overextended, the brain sends a nerve command to the muscle to contract or cramp. Flexing gradually and gently prevents spasm and tears. Only gradual movement allows full range of motion, prevents strain, and builds stamina. This allover flexibility is important because tightness in one place can cause problems and imbalances in another place.

RELAXATION MEANS NOT DOING

There are many good things you can't push, and an involuntary muscle is one of them. Of the two types of muscles, voluntary muscles can be moved at will and gain direct benefit during exercise. Involuntary muscles cannot be moved at will and only receive referred benefit from exercise when you release a contraction of a voluntary muscle. Then the involuntary muscle lengthens and returns to its starting position. You cannot act to force it to lengthen; you can only not contract.

Release and relaxation are states of physical nonaction and mental release triggered by the absence of the brain's command to act. Because exercise involves both action and nonaction of the muscles and of the brain's mental controls, there is an emotional as well as a physical aspect to all movement.

The Creator arranges everything in consideration of everything else.
—*Hildegard of Bingen*

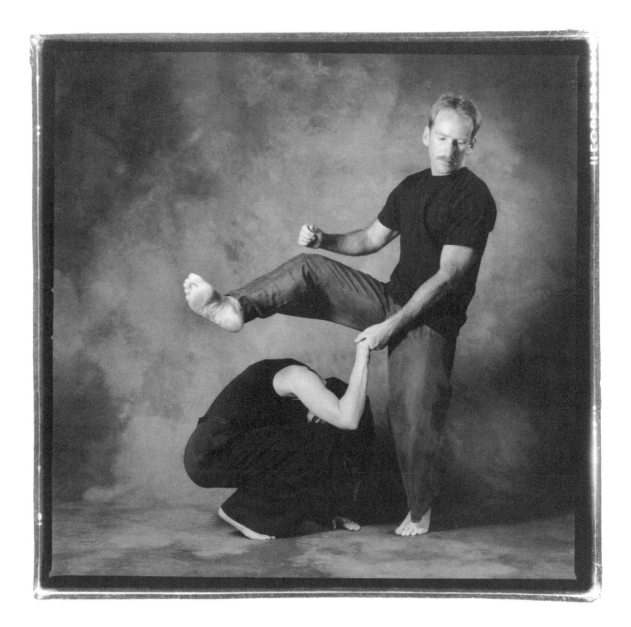

ENERGY STRETCHING

There are no miracles, only unknown laws.
—Saint Augustine

Goodness, gracious, great balls of fire!
—Jerry Lee Lewis

Our energy systems need stretching along with our muscles and bones. Energy is a valued commodity. It wouldn't occur to most of us to question whether or not energy is real just because we can't see it. We experience its effects daily. Usually we have enough steam to perform our activities, but sometimes our power is not equal to our tasks. We'd like to be able to renew our energy at will and we employ a variety of techniques in this effort. Asian disciplines can add valuable information to our Western endeavors, because they offer detailed maps of the body's energy system.

In Indian medical and spiritual terminology, the word for energy is *prana*, which is thought to come from the air we breathe. "Most of the energy for the body we get from the air we breathe, and not, as is commonly assumed, from food and water" (Swami Vishnudevananda, *The Complete Illustrated Book of Yoga*). In traditional Japanese medicine, philosophy, and martial arts, the term for energy

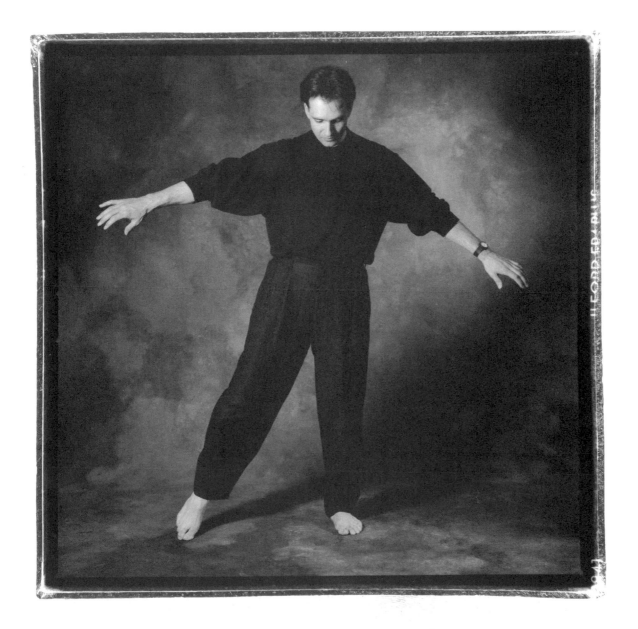

is *ki*. Chinese medicinal and spiritual systems label energy *ch'i*.

In all cultures, energy level is one index of health. In Chinese medicine, appropriate energy flow through the body is considered the most important indicator and source of good health. "Energy imbalance—its excess or insufficiency—is the root of illness; its absence is death" (Yoshio Manaka, M.D., *The Layman's Guide to Acupuncture*).

The Chinese medical system of acupuncture was developed more than four thousand years ago from observation that specific places on the body become sensitive or sore when a person is ailing. A map of these spots shows lines connecting the points that affect one another most directly. Westerners call these lines of the energy pathways "meridians." Western science acknowledges the existence of electromagnetic currents, or meridians, in the body that can affect health and can be measured by scientific equipment. The Chinese names for the negative and positive charges of electricity are *yin* and *yang*. Imbalance of these two currents in our bodies is seen as the root of all pathology.

O body swayed to music, O brightening glance
How can we know the dancer from the dance?
—William Butler Yeats

Western doctors use electrostim treatments and physical therapy to revive damaged muscles. Asian medicine uses acupuncture stimulation and exercise. *The Layman's Guide to Acupuncture* is a helpful book for practical use.

Remember that as you exercise a body part, you stimulate the energy center located there. When you are stretching your muscles, you are balancing and recharging your whole electrical energy system. By now you should be comfortable enough with your stretching to add awareness of the energy centers as you practice the exercises in the following sections.

> *As she thinks about all of life's mystery*
> *And how slowly the answers unfold,*
> *She's becoming gold.*
> —Marc Cohn

ENERGY CENTERS

The word for a biological nerve plexus, or center, in Indian yoga terminology is chakra. Each nerve center is thought to be a junction for spiritual as well as physical energy.

1. PELVIC PLEXUS: Kundalini Chakra—starting point of the body's life energy and seat of basic molecular health and balance; base of spine.

2. SEX ORGANS: Sexual Chakra—origin of erotic passion and biological creation.

3. BELLY PLEXUS: Navel Chakra—center point of physical and spiritual balance; sense of self and inner calm.

4. SOLAR PLEXUS: Action Chakra—diaphragm; channel for outer-directed power.

5. CARDIAC PLEXUS: Heart Chakra—center of compassion; can infuse all other chakras with this aspect.

6. VAGUS NERVE and CERVICAL GANGLION: Throat Chakra—communication.

7. PINEAL GLAND: Mental Chakra—third eye or center of clear, rational perception.

8. PITUITARY GLAND: Spiritual Chakra—top of head; sense of perspective and unity.

The music makes her heart belong,
The waves fall down, Nirvana waves.
—Genghis Angus

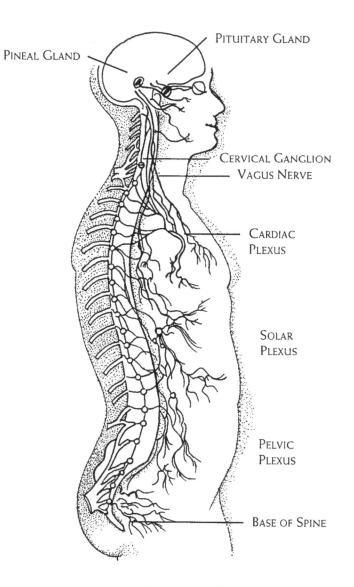

PINEAL GLAND

PITUITARY GLAND

CERVICAL GANGLION
VAGUS NERVE

CARDIAC
PLEXUS

SOLAR
PLEXUS

PELVIC
PLEXUS

BASE OF SPINE

CHAKRA ENERGY CENTERS

ACUPUNCTURE ENERGY

CENTERS

THE CHANNELS AND PRESSURE POINTS

For clarity, the diagrams on this page show the Channels on one side of the body only. All Channels except the Governor Vessel and Conception Vessel Channels are symmetrical about the midline. You will find the same points located in the same places on the opposite side of the body.

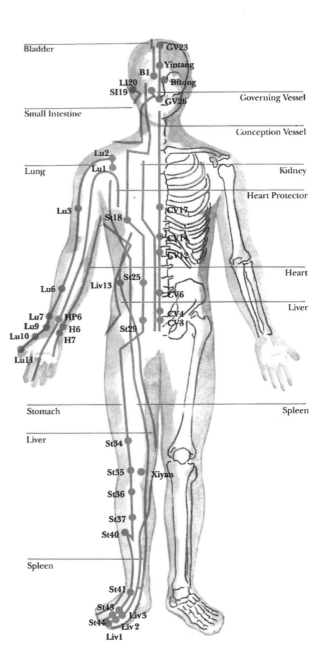

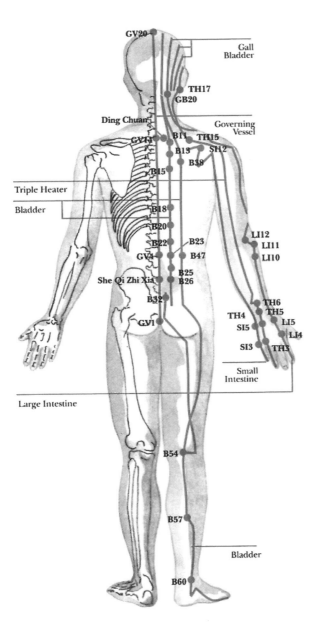

GV20

Gall
Bladder

TH17
GB20

Ding Chuan

Governing
Vessel

GV14   B11   TH15
B13   SI2
B38
B15

Triple Heater

Bladder

B18

B20

B22   B23
GV4   B47

B25
She Qi Zhi Xia   B26

B32

GV1

LI12
LI11
LI10

TH6
TH5
TH4
LI5
SI5   LI4
SI3   TH3

Small
Intestine

B54

Large Intestine

B57

Bladder

B60

Lu	Lung
LI	Large Intestine
St	Stomach
Sp	Spleen
H	Heart
SI	Small Intestine
B	Bladder
K	Kidney
HP	Heart Protector
TH	Triple Heater
GB	Gall Bladder
Liv	Liver
CV	Conception Vessel
GV	Governing Vessel

HIGH STRETCHING

Fascinatin' rhythm
You've got me on the go.
—George and Ira Gershwin

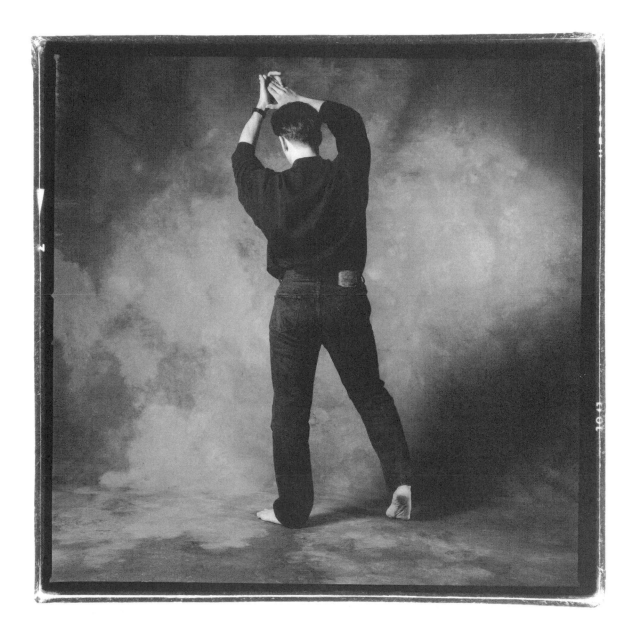

HIP TURN—RIGHT

Cowboy hula.

This stretches your hip and waist muscles and relaxes your shoulders.

1. Stand with your feet about shoulder width apart. Place your hands on your hips and look to your right.

2. Shift your weight onto your left leg with the knee slightly bent so you can tilt your right hip up a bit toward your shoulder. Bend to your right at the waist and drop your right shoulder down toward your right hip.

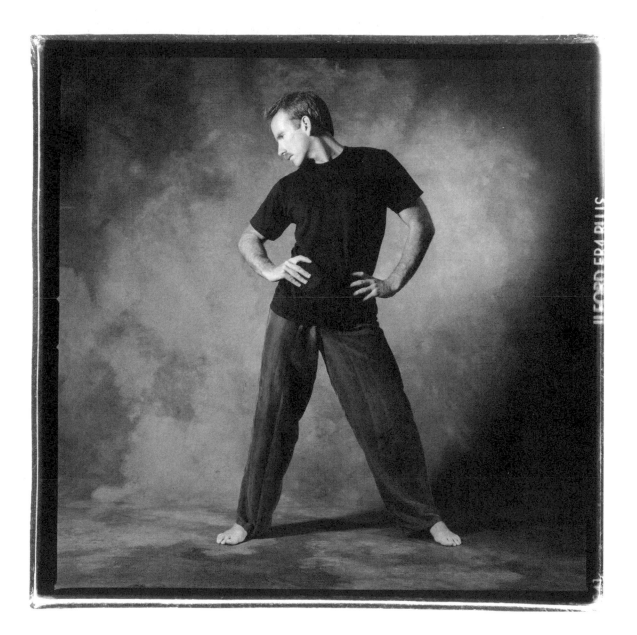

HIP TURN–MIDDLE

Elvis angles.

This movement stretches your waist, abdomen, and hip muscles.

3. Tuck your fanny under and press your pelvis forward.

4. Roll your hips from the right toward the rear until your fanny is pressed out behind you.

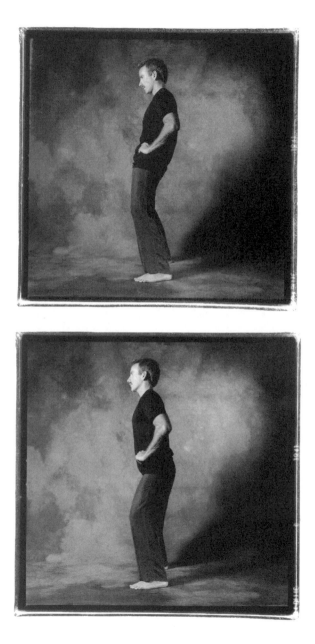

HIP TURN—LEFT

Too much.

This action relaxes your hip joints, knees, and shoulders.

5. Roll your hips to your left. Look to your left. Drop your left shoulder. Tilt your left hip up as you bend at the waist and your weight shifts to your right leg.

6. Complete the circle by rolling your hips to the center again. Face forward.

7. Do several full Hip Turns in a row with no break in between. Try to keep the movement smooth and continuous.

8. Make a full Hip Turn sequence in the opposite direction. Start by rolling hips to your left, then back, then right, then center.

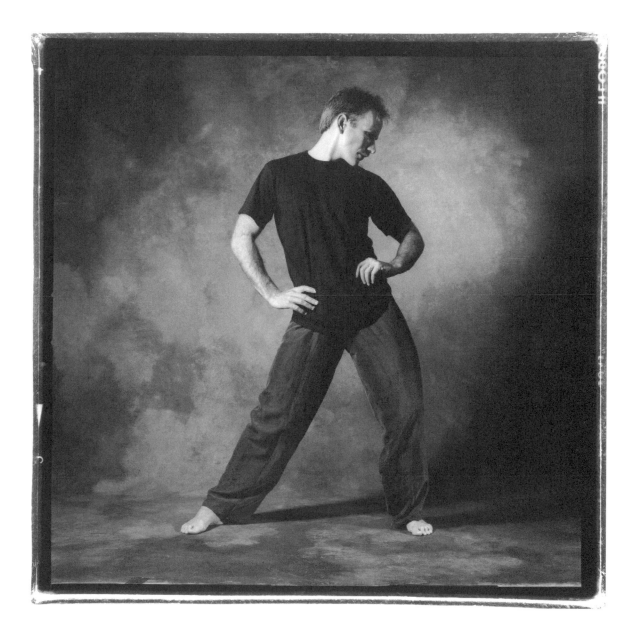

FANNY PULL

▬▬▬

Hip hop.

This movement strengthens your abdominal and pelvic muscles.

1. Place your feet about shoulder width apart. Keep your head up and forward as you press your hips back and slap both palms on your buttocks.

2. Simultaneously shove your hips forward as you press with your palms. Hop forward to a new spot on the floor.

3. Press your hips back to start the hop again.

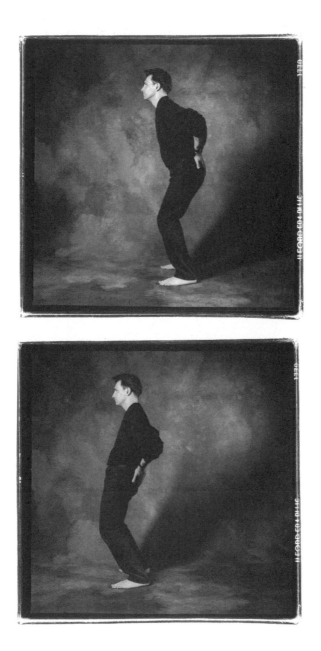

GRAPEVINE − RIGHT

A vintage stroll.

This exercise relaxes your legs and improves coordination.

1. Face forward with your feet about shoulder width apart and your arms either on your hips or stretched out to your sides, palms facing the floor. Each time you step down in this sequence, bend your knees to accentuate it. Always keep your torso facing forward to give your hips and waist more stretch.

2. Leaning to your right, step across in front of the right foot with your left leg and shift your weight to your forward left foot.

3. Draw your right foot out again to your right side and step down.

4. Cross your left foot in front of your right and step onto your left foot. You can hop as you step, for variation. Continue this sequence as you move across the floor to your right in a straight line.

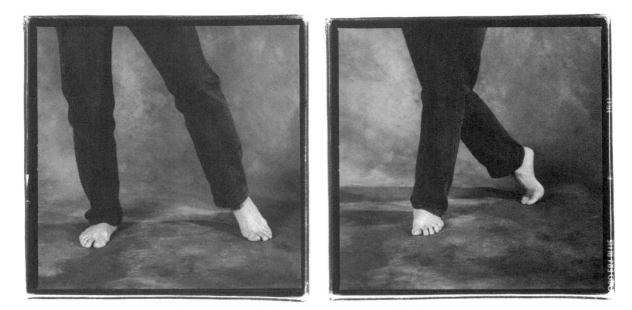
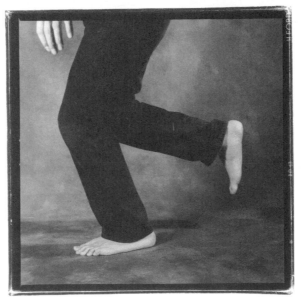

GRAPEVINE–LEFT

It's time.

5. Draw your left foot across the floor to your left. Then step and shift your weight onto your left foot.

6. With your right leg, step in front of your left foot and shift your weight to your forward right foot.

7. Draw your left foot out again to your left side and step down.

8. Cross your right foot in front of your left and step onto your right foot. You can hop as you step. Continue this sequence to move across the floor to your left in a straight line.

9. While moving in one direction, alternate cross-stepping in front of the stationary leg and next in back of it. This variation allows you to stretch your hips and waist more. You can shift directions at will.

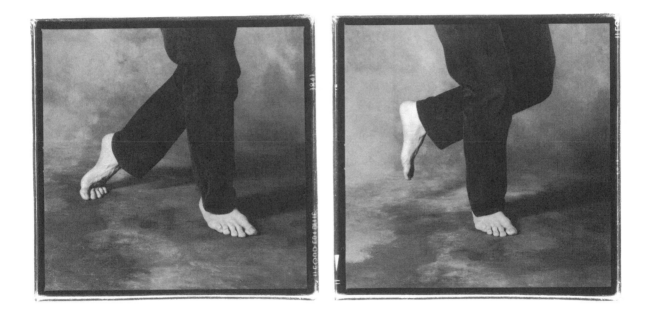

HOOK TURNS

Can be addictive.

This motion does your leg and lower back muscles a good turn.

1. Stand on your left leg. Bend your right knee and wrap your right foot behind your left knee.

2. Bend your left knee slightly as you grip your left leg with your right toes. Press and swing your right knee out to the right side and pivot a quarter turn on the ball of your left foot. You'll stop facing to the right of where you started.

3. Pivot again a quarter turn so you stop facing backward. Pivot again a quarter turn so you stop facing left. Pivot once more
a quarter turn so you finish, facing front, as you began.

4. Switch legs so your left foot is tucked behind your right knee and you are standing on your right leg. Do Hook Turns to your left.

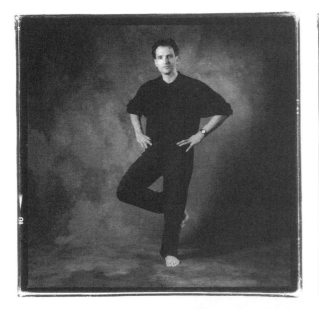
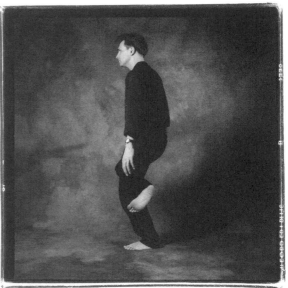
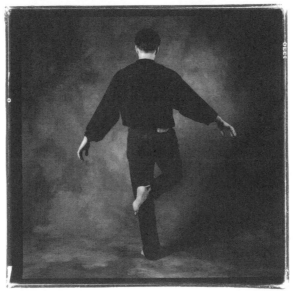

SIDE CLAPS

High hands.

This movement improves coordination and stretches arm and leg muscles.

1. Lean toward your left as you put your weight on your left leg. Raise your hands over your head and clap.

2. Swing your right leg in front of you, and then left with enough force to spin yourself around in a full circle.

3. When you have spun to the front and center again, step on your right foot. Lean right, raise your arms above your head, and clap your hands. Then try this sequence spinning to your right.

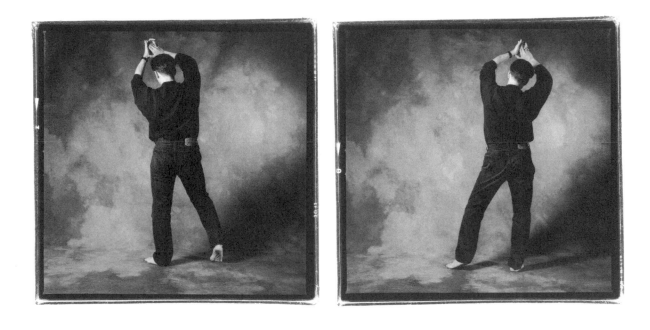

SLIDE HOP TAP

███████

Low jangles.

This movement strengthens your calf muscles.

1. Stand on your right leg with your left leg and foot stretched out to your left, toes touching the floor.

2. Bend the left knee and slide your left pointed toes along the floor until they touch your right ankle. Raise the foot several inches off the ground while touching your right leg.

3. Hop in place on your right foot.

4. Brusquely tap the toes of your left foot on the floor and raise them quickly back up beside your right leg.

5. Step down and transfer your weight onto your left leg.

6. Raise your right heel off the ground, bending your right knee. Slide your right foot out to your right to begin the Slide Hop Tap sequence to the other side.

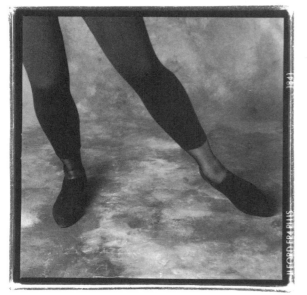
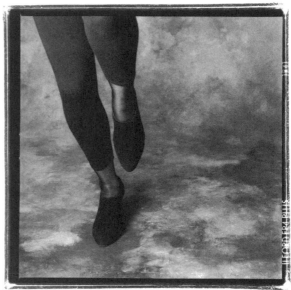
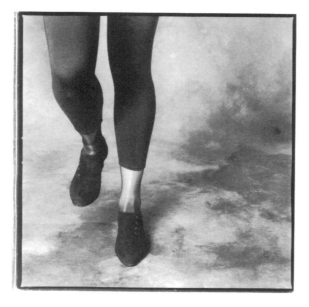

FLAPPER KNEES

Charleston tradition.

This motion helps keep your knee and thigh muscles flexible.

1. Place your feet about shoulder width apart. Press both knees outward to the sides, away from each other.

2. Keeping your feet stationary, draw both knees in until they touch.

3. Press both knees outward again. Alternate directions several times.

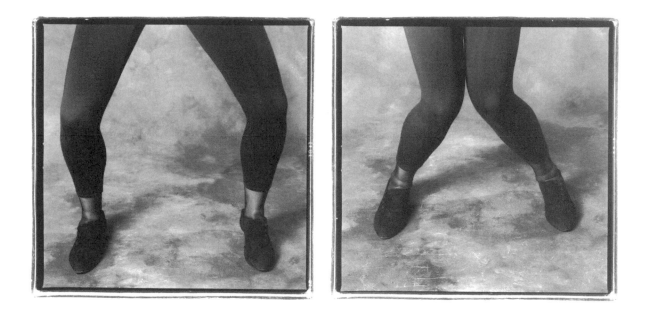

FLOOR PAT—RIGHT

Get down.

This stretches your back, arm, and leg muscles.

1. Stand facing forward with your legs shoulder width apart. Look to your right as you turn and lean your torso to the right. Keep your right arm against your right side. Stretch your left leg out to the left.

2. Bend your right knee as deeply as is comfortable.

3. Keep your head up as you bring your left palm down to touch the floor in front of your right foot.

4. Return to center by standing up.

If you do this exercise slowly, hold the stretch for a while. If you want to do it faster, just tap the floor and return to center.

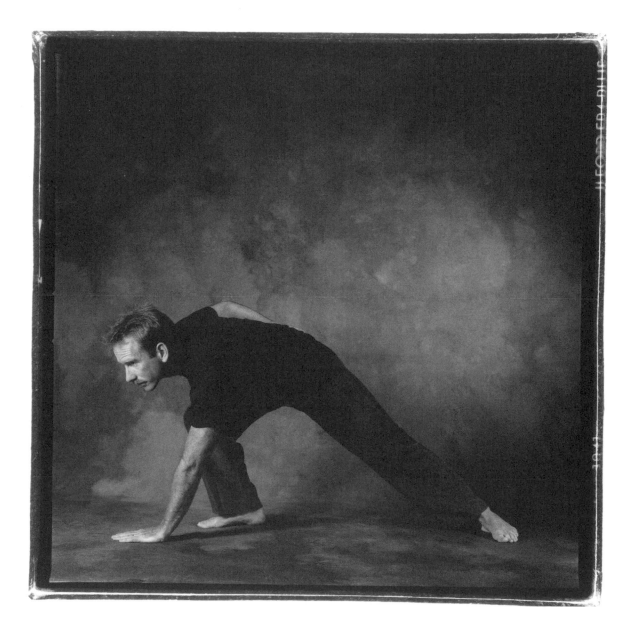

FLOOR PAT—LEFT

Touch the earth.

5. Stand facing forward. Turn your head to your left. Bend your left knee and lean to your left. Keep your left arm straight against your left side.

6. Slide your right leg out to your right as you bring your right arm in front of you.

7. Press the palm of your right hand against the floor in front of your left foot.

8. Alternate right and left Floor Pats. Stand up in the center in between each. Try to make the movement smooth.

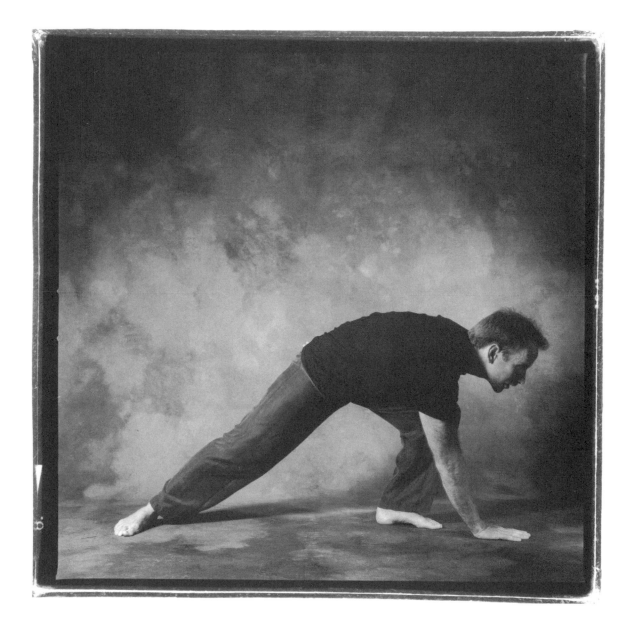

HOP CLAP

Applaud yourself.

This movement relaxes the leg, foot, and arm muscles.

1. Step on your right leg. Hop as you raise your left leg with knee bent and toes flexed. Clap.

2. Reverse the action and Hop Clap on your left leg.

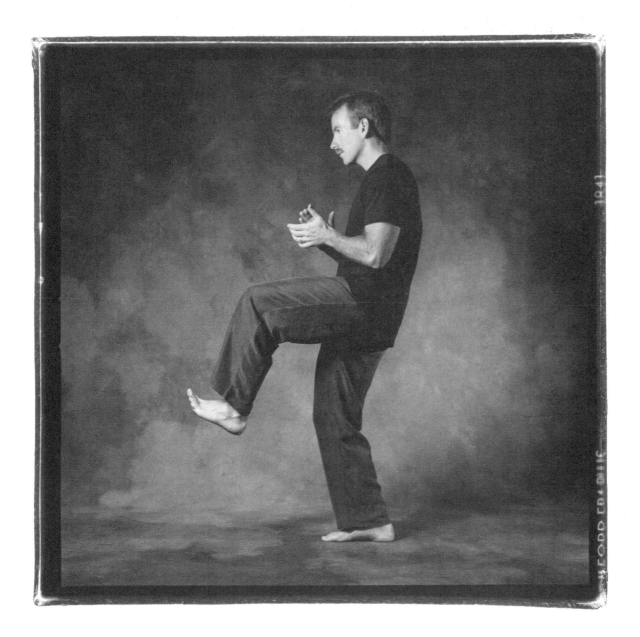

TWO STRETCH

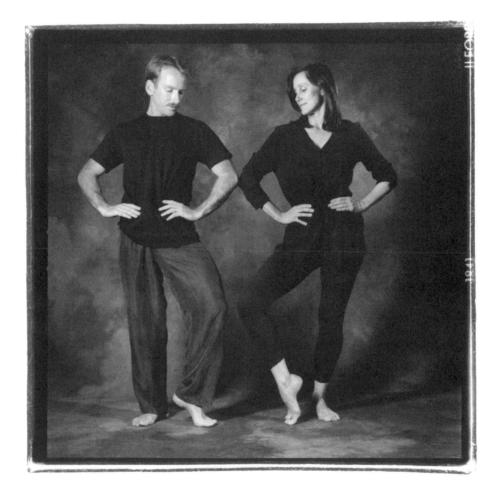

FLEXIBLE PARTNERSHIPS
TWO STRETCH

IV

TWO STRETCH

FLEXIBLE PARTNERSHIPS

Dance with me; I want my arms about you;
The charms about you will carry me through.
—*Irving Berlin*

Stretching does not have to be a solitary meditation. It can be reciprocal relaxation. The photos show a man and woman, but any two people can do these exercises for fun and relaxation. How two people work and play together mirrors the rest of their patterns of interaction. You can ease emotional as well as physical tension by learning to play together. It is also very satisfying to achieve a mutual goal while supporting each other.

Many of the stretches in this section are only possible and become more interesting when done together. The way you interact when learning and problem solving can also be enlightening and pleasurable. You may understand things about yourselves that you wouldn't see another way, and you'll improve your nonverbal communication. When you're in a close relationship, there are lots of things that you can do alone, but it takes two to untangle.

EGYPTIAN HANDS

A palm date.

1. To establish your basic position, stand side by side with one person slightly behind the other. Relax your breathing so you can feel a slight movement in the muscles of your belly as you inhale and exhale. Position your feet facing forward, a small distance apart so you stand firmly. Bend the knees a bit.

2. The man's right arm is stretched out to his right side, while his left arm is held close to his left side.

3. If the woman is to the man's right, keeping her elbows bent, she places her downturned left palm on top of his upturned left palm, just below shoulder height. Her right palm is upturned to face his downturned right palm.

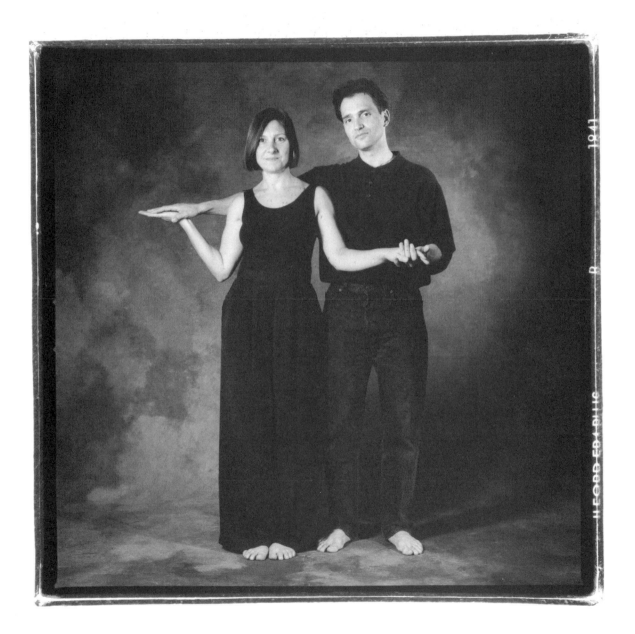

DOUBLE KNEE BENDS — RIGHT

Walk like an Egyptian.

These steps are performed in unison. Walk through the sequence in slow motion to start. Then speed up the tempo as you feel comfortable. The moves strengthen all your muscles.

1. Keep your torsos facing forward and arms in position at about shoulder height.

2. The man turns his hips to his right and steps with his left leg to the front and across his right foot. He deepens the knee bend as he steps down.

3. At the same time the woman swings her left leg in front of her right and brings her left foot across in front of her right leg, deepening her knee bends as she steps down.

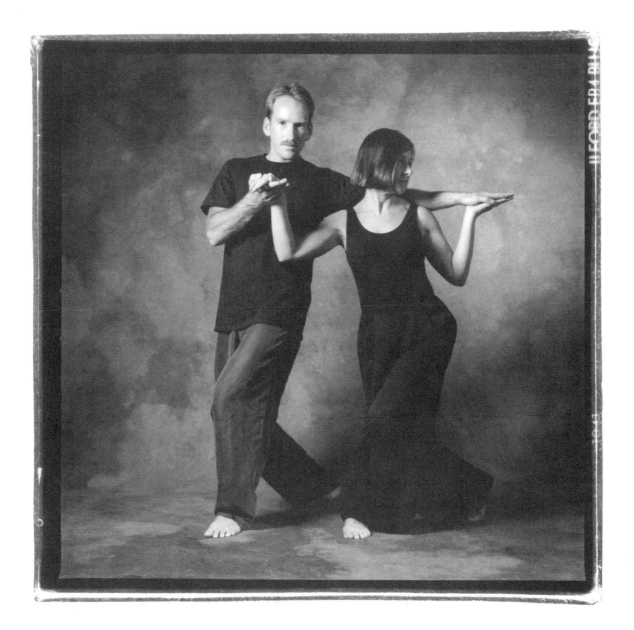

DOUBLE KNEE BENDS — LEFT

■■■■■■■

Tut strut.

4. Both people shift their weight and step back onto the left foot while straightening the left leg.

5. Bring the left leg back to step beside the right foot.

6. Pick up the right foot and step down in place.

7. Turn the hips toward the left. The man steps down onto his left foot. Then he swings his right leg in front of his left and steps down with knees bent, forward onto his right foot.

8. Simultaneously the woman swings her right leg across her left and steps down onto her right foot.

9. Both people step back onto their rear feet. Then both bring the forward legs back to step down beside that foot to end in the center position as they began.

10. Repeat this whole sequence at least twice to each side.

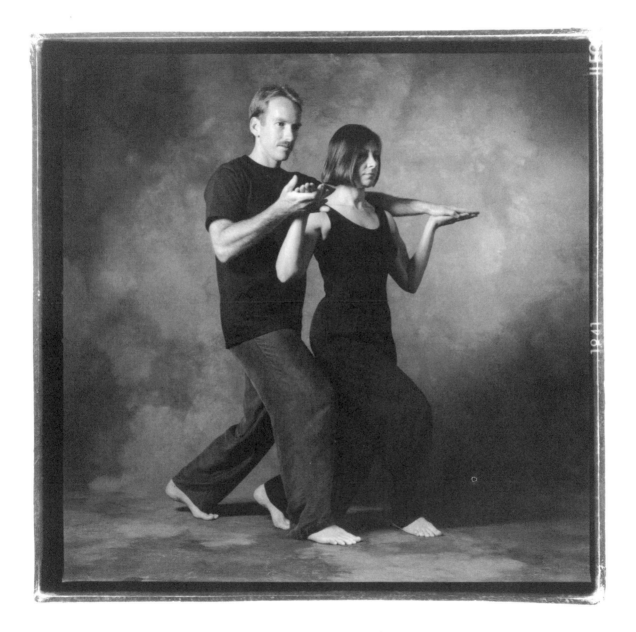

TUT STOP

▬▬▬

Frieze.

1. In unison, shift weight onto one leg. Point the toe of the other foot forward and tap it twice on the floor in front of you.

2. Hop in place once on the rear foot.

3. Bring the forward foot beside the rear foot and step down to shift weight onto it as you raise the opposite leg off the ground. Repeat this tapping sequence with the other leg pointing to the opposite side.

4. As you feel more limber, you can raise your tapping leg higher until the motion becomes a kick. Repeat on both sides.

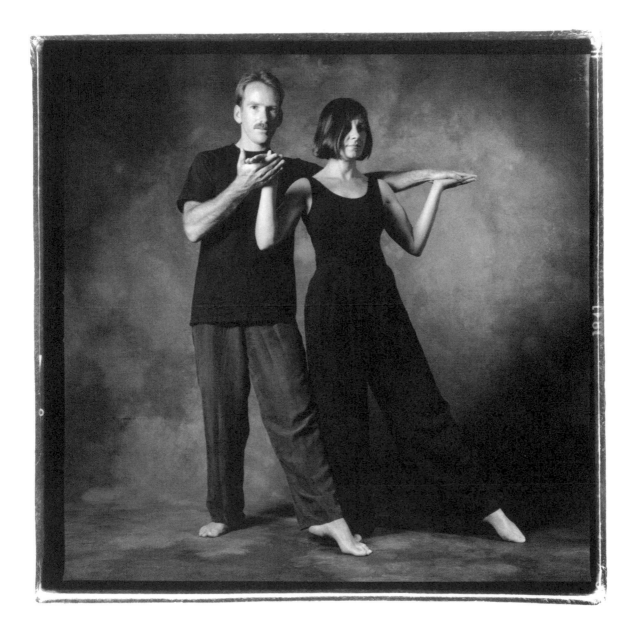

KNEE CIRCLES—OUT

Don't knock knees.

This motion flexes the knee joints, thighs, and ankles.

1. Stay in the same spot on the floor while standing side by side with your hands on your hips and your feet about shoulder width apart. Shift your weight onto your inside leg. Facing forward, you bend the knee of the outside leg.

2. Keeping the toes on the floor, roll your bent knee outward so it gives the thigh a good stretch. Press back with the thigh muscles and roll the bent knee back in beside your straight leg to end as you began.

3. Repeat this motion forward, out, and back again as though you are drawing circles in the air with your knee. Draw four circles in this direction.

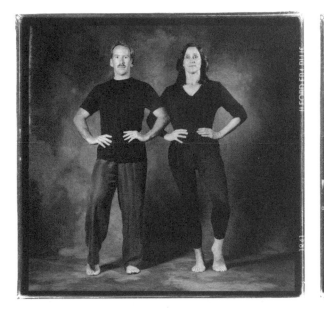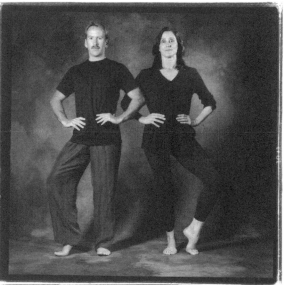

KNEE CIRCLES—IN

Will the circle be unbroken?

4. Shift your weight so you are standing on your outside leg. The heel of your inside leg is now off the floor. Point your bent inside knee toward your partner's knee. Push your inside thigh outward and back. Now roll your inside knee back toward your straight leg to end as you began.

5. Keeping your toes on the ground, repeat this motion so that you draw four circles in the air with your inside knee.

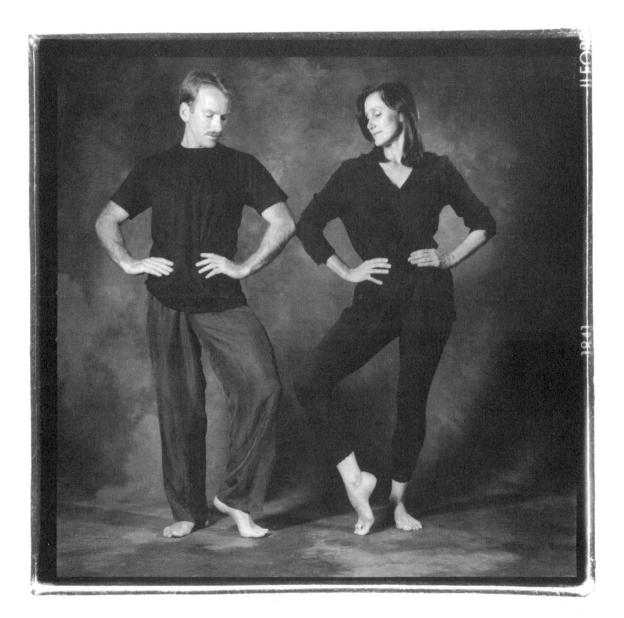

SHOULDER SHIMMY

■

All shook up.

This movement relaxes the torso and shoulders.

1. If you are standing side by side, swing your outside leg a half circle toward your inside leg until you spin to a position facing one another. Your knees are bent and your hips are pushed back. Form light fists. Turn your head to the right.

2. Keeping your head and hips stationary, shake your upper torso and shoulders from side to side. Practice slowly at first; then speed up until the motion qualifies as a bona fide shimmy.

3. You can shift your weight now and then from foot to foot to add more movement and rhythm to your shimmy.

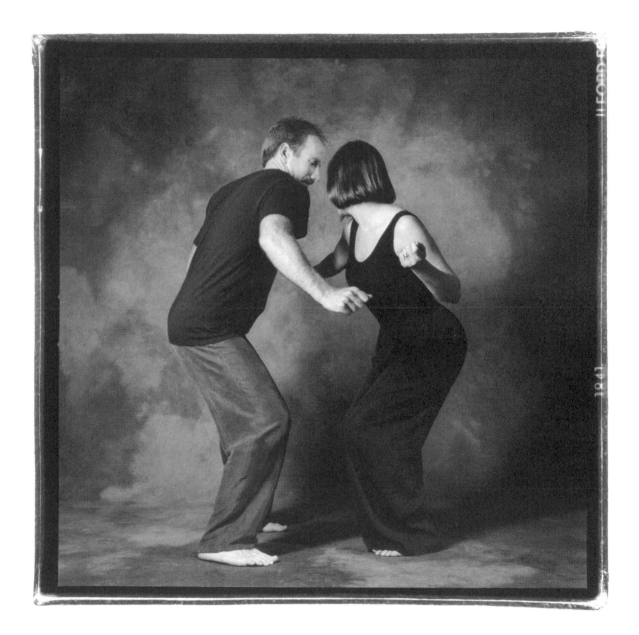

HIP SHIMMY

All shook down.

This motion relaxes the lower back and hip muscles.

1. Face forward. Keep your knees bent. Place both palms at your waist or on your hips behind you. Push your hips back and your chest forward.

2. Keep your torso and feet stationary while you move your hips from left to right. Move slowly at first, and then speed up so you are shaking your hips from side to side as fast as you can.

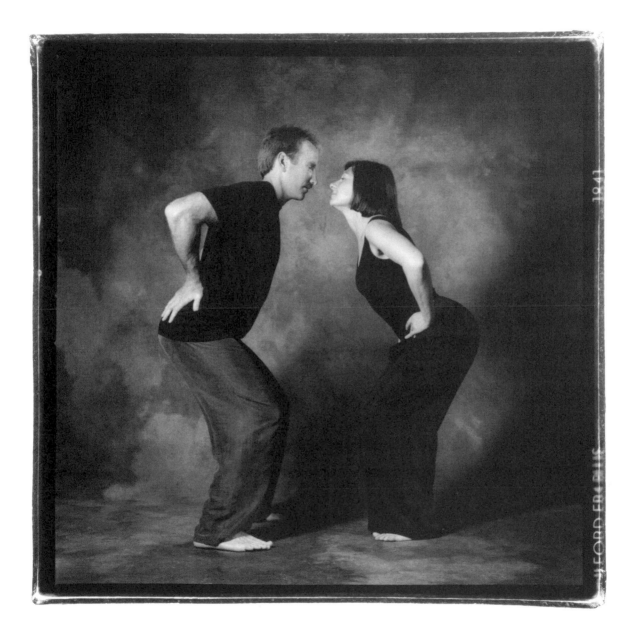

MOON RISE—START

It's only...

This movement sequence stretches almost all your muscles in almost every direction they move.

1. Clasp hands between you. Tilt your pelvis forward and relax your chest.

2. Shift your weight so you are standing on your outside leg (the man's right; the woman's left).

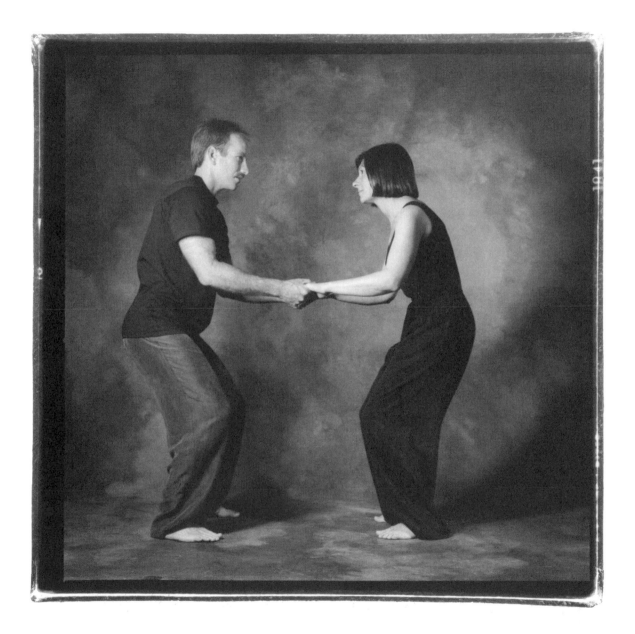

MOON RISE

▃▃▃▃

A paper moon...

The following steps are described separately, but should be performed simultaneously so they form a complete sweeping motion.

3. Raise your outside arm (the man's right; the woman's left) high up over your head as you lower your inside arm.

4. At the same time, turn your torso and head forward. The man turns to his right; the woman turns to her left. Also swing your inside leg forward between the two of you so you are both standing facing outward now.

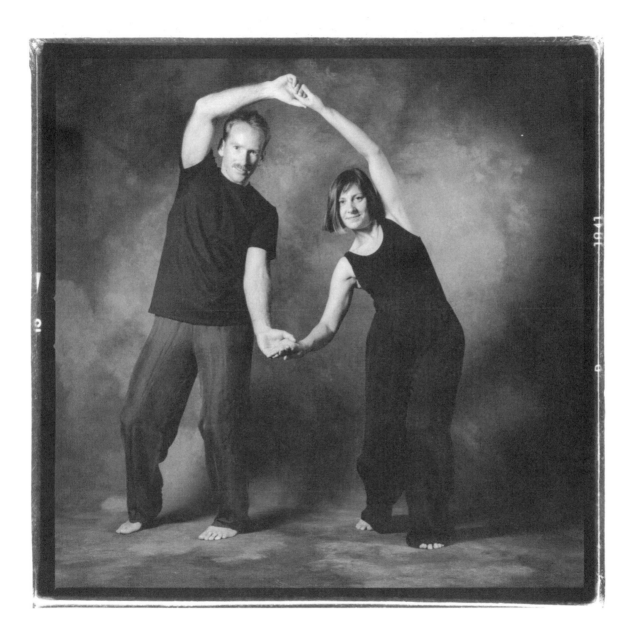

FULL MOON

Sailing over a cardboard sea...

5. Continue to turn in the same outward direction while keeping your hands clasped together.

6. End up back to back, arching backward and keeping your hands clasped. The palms are now facing up.

7. Raise your arms as high as is comfortable as you tilt your pelvis forward to accentuate the arch.

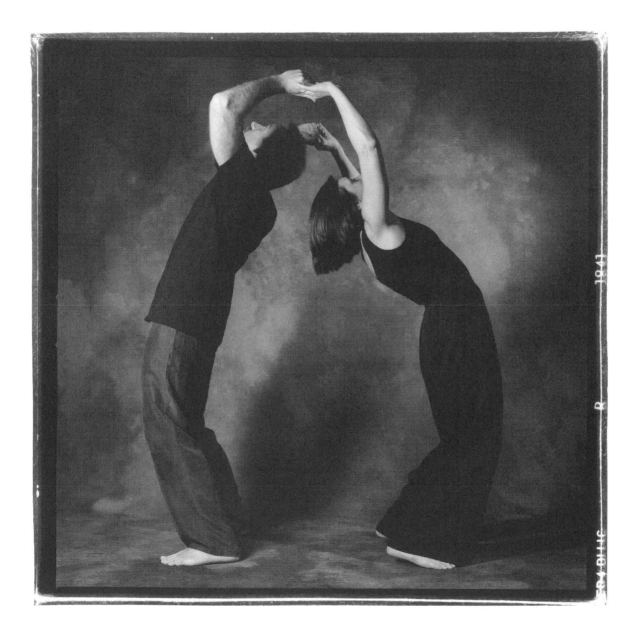

MOON SET

But it wouldn't be make-believe
If you believed in me.
—Rose & Harburg

8. Continue to step and turn in the same direction while maintaining clasped hands.

9. Roll down out of the arch by stepping to the opposite side (man to his right; woman to her left), until you have your outside arms (man's left; woman's right) overhead and your inside arms down at your sides between you.

10. Gradually complete the turn so that you come full circle back to your starting position, facing one another.

You can rest in the center a moment. Or you can keep moving so that you being in the Moon Rise all over again without pausing. Practice this slowly. Speed up the pace so that you can perform four full Moon Rises in a row.

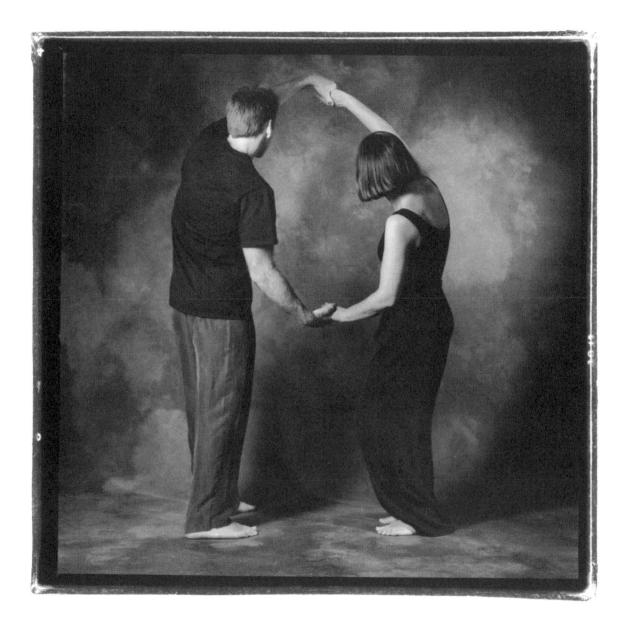

SHOULDER 8

You've got a hold on me.

This sequence stretches neck, arm, chest, and shoulder muscles.

1. Facing your partner with hands clasped, step toward each other with your right feet so that your torsos are facing in opposite directions, but you are looking at one another.

2. At the same time, raise your arms above your head so you can slip into the following position: Straighten your right arms and rest the clasped hands on the back of your partner's neck. Simultaneously bend your left elbow so you can reach the figure 8 arm position behind the head.

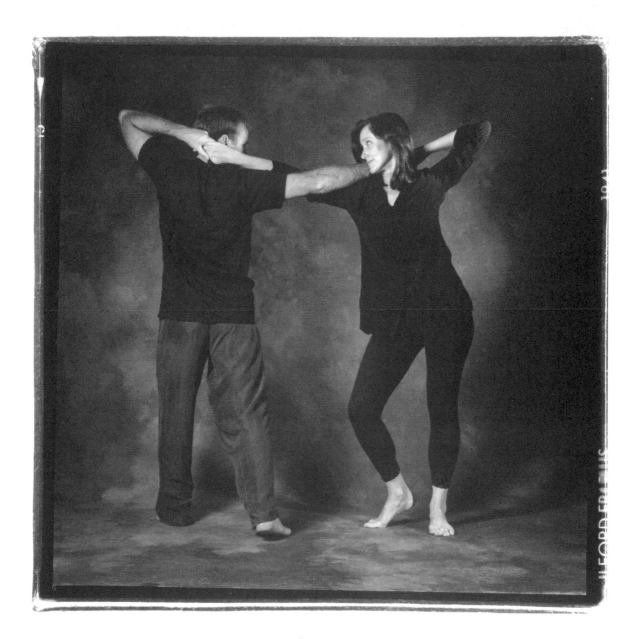

SHOULDER 8 SLIDE

Don't let go.

3. Release your outside hands and arms and relax them at your sides. Keep your inside hands clasped.

4. Lean backward while maintaining a firm grip on your clasped right arms for support.

5. Slide your hand grip down from the shoulder toward the wrist. At the same time, lengthen this slide by moving your feet away from your partner in a Pigeon (page 22).

6. End the slide with clasped palms. You can move into a turn or into the next position by releasing your arms and making a full spin in place until you're facing one another again. Or you can simply clasp your hands in front of you as you began.

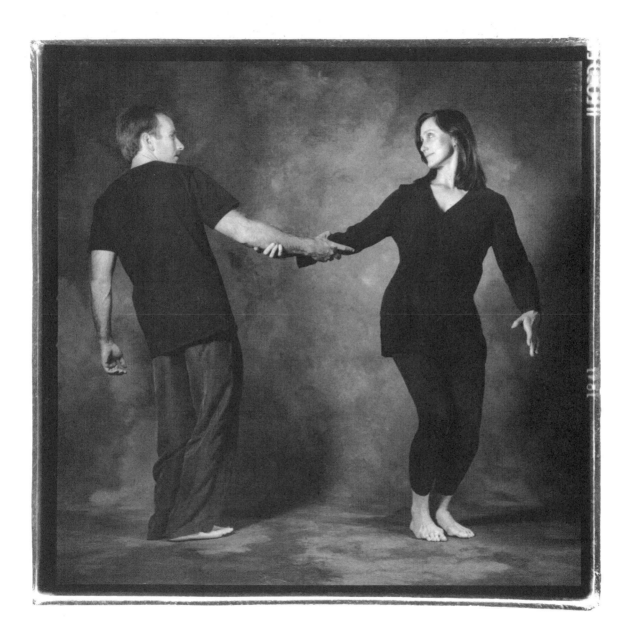

THREAD THE NEEDLE – START

I wanna hold your hand.

This sequence improves coordination and stretches almost all your muscles.

1. Draw your clasped hands close together between you. Establish a firm grip. The man stands upright. The woman steps backward to allow about two feet of space between them.

2. The woman bends her knees more so she can lower herself into a squatting position while maintaining clasped hands.

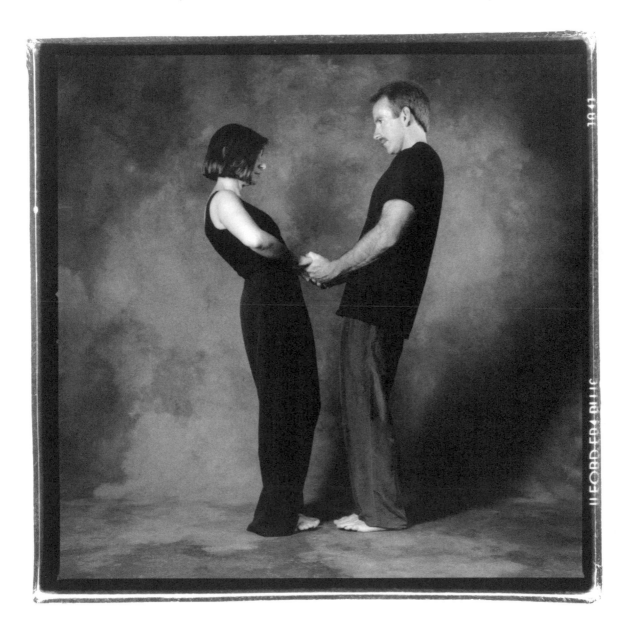

THREAD THE NEEDLE – KNEEL

You're the top.

3. The standing person straightens his arms to allow the partner to sink into a crouching position in front of him.

4. She keeps a firm grip on his hands as she tucks her head forward and bends her arms.

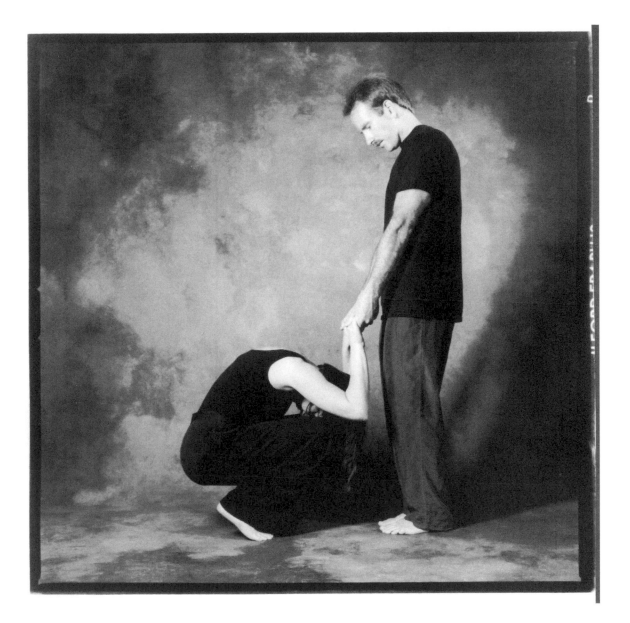

THREAD THE NEEDLE-KICK

My heart stood still.

5. The kneeling person lets go of the standing person's right hand so she can steady herself with her left hand on the floor.

6. The kneeling person leans her torso down and curls forward as tight as possible, making sure to keep her head very low.

7. The standing person shifts his weight onto his left leg as he raises his right leg. He swings his whole body around in a half circle to his left with the force from the leg motion. He kicks high above the crouching person's back and swings his right leg to the other side (her right side) of the kneeling person. You will probably have to kick slowly at first and work up to a fast kick with practice.

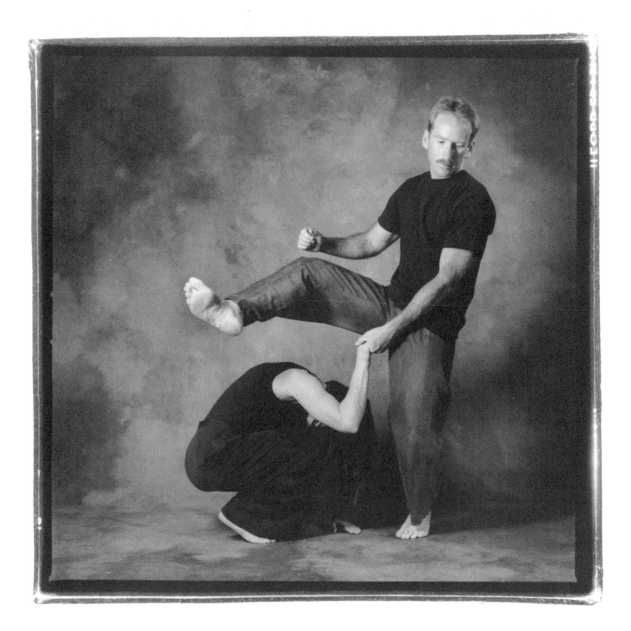

THREAD THE NEEDLE-TUG

Jeepers creepers.

8. He ends standing and bent forward with his back to the kneeling person.

9. He clasps both her hands in his as she reaches forward between his legs. The grasp is firm, and they are leaning away from one another to help support each other's positions.

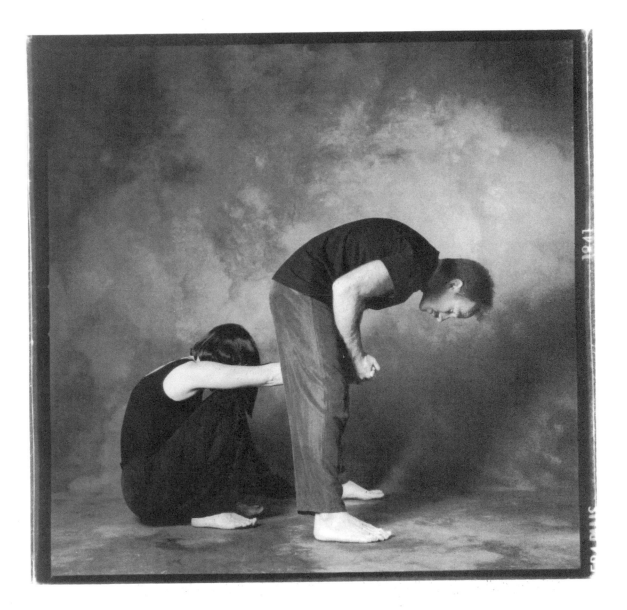

THREAD THE NEEDLE—THROUGH

Bravo.

10. The standing person widens his stance so his feet are more than shoulder width apart. The standing person draws the kneeling person's hands forward through his legs as he begins to stand up straight.

11. The kneeling person walks forward in the crouched position through the standing person's legs until she is in front of him.

12. The standing person's arms are stretched out taut in front of him while the kneeling person's arms are reaching upward in front of her. The grip is firm for mutual support.

13. He pulls her up until she is standing in front of him.

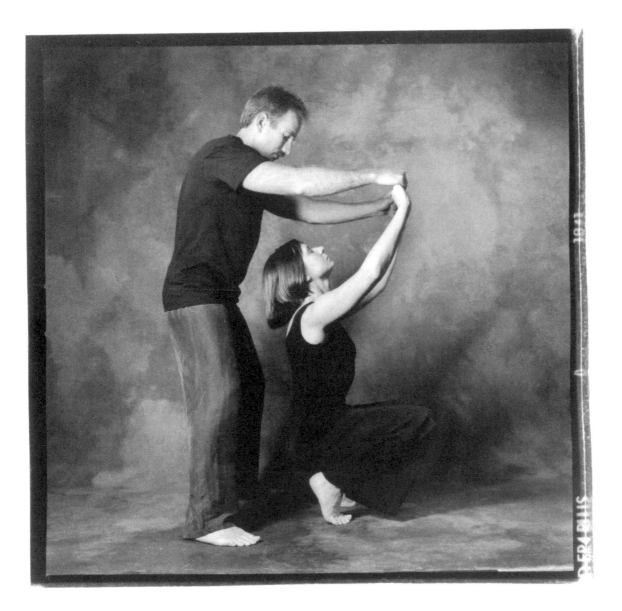

TWO REST

Who could ask for anything more?

1. At the close of Thread the Needle (page 172), she does a full turn to her left toward him. She ends with her back to him.

2. She crosses her arms so he can grab her hands on either side. They both lean back slightly, pointing their right legs forward and resting comfortably against one another.

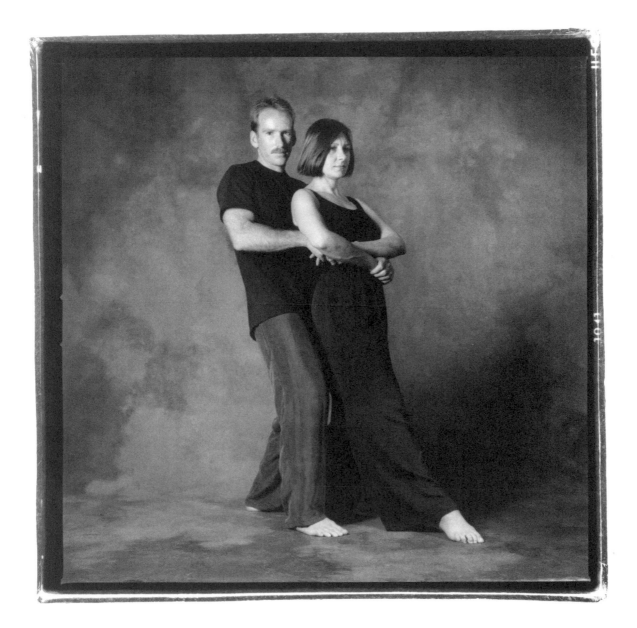

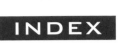

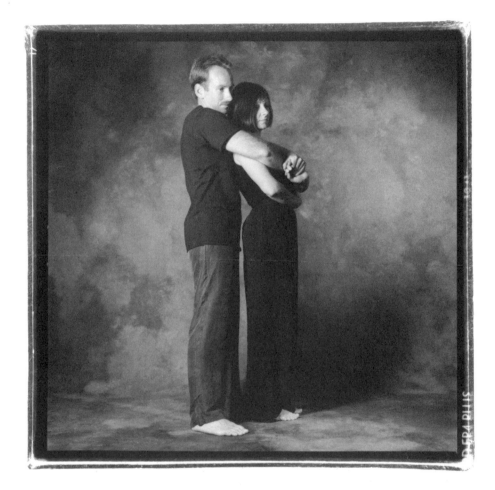

SPORT STRETCHES
THE EXERCISES

INDEX

SPORT STRETCHES

BASEBALL/SOFTBALL/HOCKEY: Shoulder Snakes, Pigeon, Squat Rest, Lily, Visualization, Leg Leans, Step Slide Hop, Hip Turns, Side Claps, Slide Hop Tap, Flapper Knees, Floor Pats, Double Knee Bends, Knee Circles, Shoulder 8.

BASKETBALL/VOLLEYBALL/LACROSSE: Shoulder Snakes, Elbow Hip Flip, Foot Fans, Pigeon, Side Hops, Basic Breath, Neck Release, Full Spine Release, Frog Flex, Squat Rest, Visualization, Breathe For Action, Palm Sphere, Leg Leans, Body Pull, Heel Rock, Sole Slap, Step Slide Hop, Hip Turns, Grapevine, Side Claps, Flapper Knees, Hop Claps, Knee Circles, Shoulder Shimmy, Moon Cycle.

FOOTBALL/RUGBY: Shoulder Snakes, Heel Stomps, Elbow Hip Flip, Neck Release, Full Spine Release, Frog Flex, Squat Rest, Lily, Visualization, Breathe For Action, Long Leg Leans, Body Pull, Hip Slap, Hip Turns, Fanny Pull, Flapper Knees, Floor Pats, Hip Shimmy, Shoulder 8.

GOLF: Cleopatra Roll, Shoulder Snakes, Elbow Hip Flip, Foot Fans, Basic Breath, Neck Release, Full Spine Release, Egg Ball, Squat Rest, Visualization, Breathe For Action, Palm Sphere, Leg Rock, Hip Slap, Energy Stretching, Hip Turns, Knee Circles, Moon Cycle, Shoulder 8.

GYMNASTICS/DANCE/SKATING/SURFING/MARTIAL ARTS: Cleopatra Roll, Shoulder Snakes, Side Hops, Heel Stomps, Basic Breath, Neck Release, Full Spine Release, Frog Flex, Egg Ball, Squat Rest, Lily, Back Rest, Visualization, Breathe For Action, Palm Sphere, Leg Leans, Heel Rock, Sole Slap, Step Slide Hop, Energy Stretching, Hip Turns, Fanny Pull, Grapevine, Hook Turns, Flapper Knees, Floor Pats, Double Knee Bends, Moon Cycle, Thread the Needle.

POLO/RIDING: Cleopatra Roll, Shoulder Snakes, Foot Fans, Basic Breath, Full Spine Release, Frog Flex, Egg Ball, Squat Rest, Lily, Visualization, Breathe For Action, Palm Sphere, Hip Slap, Energy Stretching, Hip Turns, Flapper Knees, Floor Pats, Moon Cycle, Shoulder 8.

RUNNING: Shoulder Snakes, Foot Fans, Heel Stomps, Basic Breath, Frog Flex, Egg Ball, Squat Rest, Lily, Back Rest, Visualization, Breathe For Action, Leg Rock, Leg Leans, Heel Rock, Step Slide Hop, Energy Stretching, Hip Turns, Grapevine, Hook Turns, Flapper Knees, Hop Claps.

SOCCER/HIKING: Cleopatra Roll, Shoulder Snakes, Foot Fans, Pigeon, Heel Stomps, Basic Breath, Neck Release, Frog Flex, Squat Rest, Lily, Visualization, Breathe For Action, Leg Rock, Leg Leans, Hip Slap, Heel Rock, Sole Slap, Step Slide Hop, Energy Stretching, Hip Turns, Hooks Turns, Flapper Knees, Thread the Needle.

SKIING/CYCLING: Shoulder Snakes, Elbow Hip Flip, Pigeon, Side Hops, Basic Breath, Full Spine Release, Frog Flex, Egg Ball, Lily, Visualization, Breathe For Action, Leg Rocks, Leg Leans, Hip Slap, Heel Rock, Sole Slap, Energy Stretching, Hip Turns, Grapevine, Hook Turns, Flapper Knees, Double Knee Bends, Knee Circles.

SWIMMING/WATER POLO: Cleopatra Roll, Shoulder Snakes, Basic Breath, Neck Release, Full Spine Release, Visualization, Breathe For Action, Moon Cycle, Shoulder 8.

TENNIS/RACQUETBALL/SQUASH: Shoulder Snakes, Pigeon, Heel Stomp, Side Hops, Basic Breath, Full Spine Release, Squat Rest, Visualization, Breathe For Action, Leg Rock, Body Pull, Heel Rock, Sole Slap, Hip Turns, Hook Turns, Floor Pats, Moon Cycle, Thread the Needle.

WRESTLING/WEIGHT TRAINING: Cleopatra Roll, Shoulder Snakes, Basic Breath, Neck Release, Full Spine Release, Frog Flex, Squat Rest, Lily, Visualization, Breath For Action, Leg Leans, Energy Stretching, Hip Turns, Shoulder Shimmy, Hip Shimmy, Shoulder 8.

If there's no dancing at the revolution, I won't come.
—*Emma Goldman*

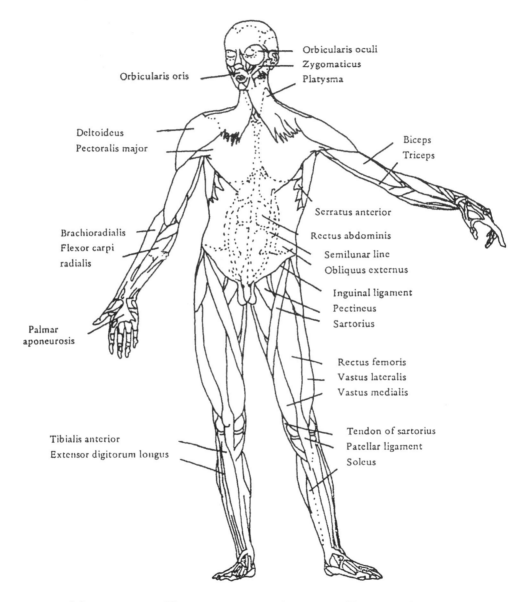

Orbicularis oculi
Zygomaticus
Platysma

Orbicularis oris

Deltoideus
Pectoralis major

Biceps
Triceps

Brachioradialis
Flexor carpi
radialis

Serratus anterior

Rectus abdominis

Semilunar line
Obliquus externus

Inguinal ligament
Pectineus
Sartorius

Palmar
aponeurosis

Rectus femoris
Vastus lateralis
Vastus medialis

Tendon of sartorius
Patellar ligament
Soleus

Tibialis anterior
Extensor digitorum longus

MUSCLES, SUPERFICIAL LAYER, FRONT VIEW

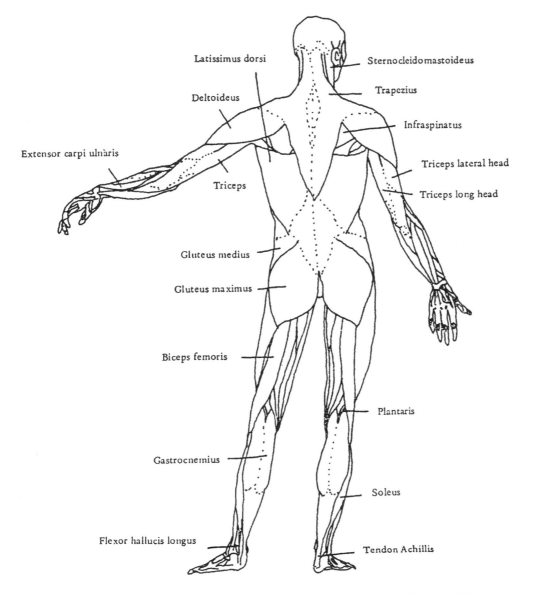

Latissimus dorsi

Deltoideus

Extensor carpi ulnaris

Triceps

Gluteus medius

Gluteus maximus

Biceps femoris

Gastrocnemius

Flexor hallucis longus

Sternocleidomastoideus

Trapezius

Infraspinatus

Triceps lateral head

Triceps long head

Plantaris

Soleus

Tendon Achillis

MUSCLES, SUPERFICIAL LAYER, BACK VIEW

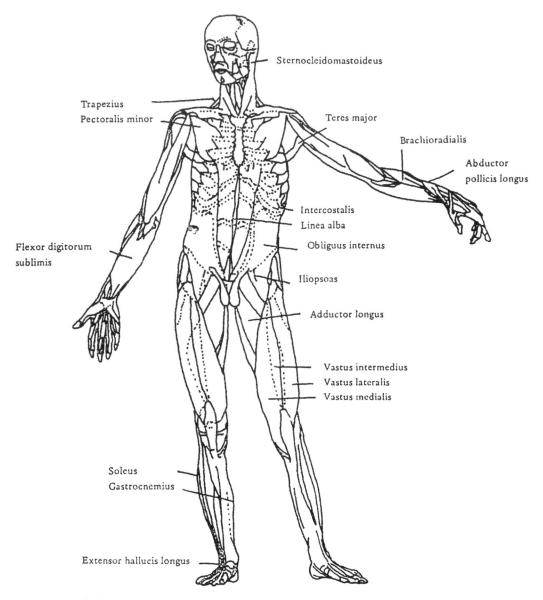

Sternocleidomastoideus

Trapezius
Pectoralis minor

Teres major

Brachioradialis

Abductor
pollicis longus

Intercostalis
Linea alba

Obliguus internus

Flexor digitorum
sublimis

Iliopsoas

Adductor longus

Vastus intermedius
Vastus lateralis
Vastus medialis

Soleus
Gastrocnemius

Extensor hallucis longus

MUSCLES, DEEP LAYER, FRONT VIEW

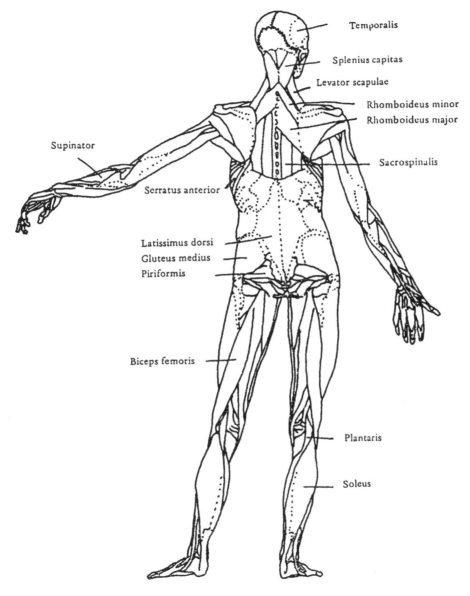

Temporalis

Splenius capitas

Levator scapulae

Rhomboideus minor

Rhomboideus major

Supinator

Sacrospinalis

Serratus anterior

Latissimus dorsi

Gluteus medius

Piriformis

Biceps femoris

Plantaris

Soleus

MUSCLES, DEEP LAYER, BACK VIEW

THE EXERCISES

TWO STRETCH

You are the sunshine of my life.
—Stevie Wonder

ACKNOWLEDGMENTS

Kudos to the flexible models:

Greg Lewis
Susan Orzel
Eugene Ruffolo
Anne Kent Rush
Dana Spot

Many thanks for special editorial help to:
Freude Bartlett, Susie Glickman, and Dottie Dunnam.

Bravo to Dinah Dunn and Amy Chisam
for their continuous support in production.

Appreciation to Kenneth Lo
for beautiful book design.

Gratitude for stretching lessons to:
Tashi Fang Wong, Pumpkin, Chip, and S'More.

Much admiration to Pat Harbron
for making the photographs so fabulous.

BOOKS BY ANNE KENT RUSH

ROMANTIC MASSAGE (Avon)

THE BACK RUB BOOK (Vintage)

THE MODERN BOOK OF YOGA (Dell)

THE MODERN BOOK OF MASSAGE (Dell)

GETTING CLEAR: BODY WORK FOR WOMEN
(Random House)

FEMINISM AS THERAPY; with Mander (Random House)

MOON, MOON (Random House–Moon Books)

GRETA BEAR GOES TO YELLOWSTONE NATIONAL PARK
(Greta Bear Enterprizes)

THE BASIC BACK BOOK (Summit/Simon & Schuster)

THE MASSAGE BOOK, by George Downing,
illustrated by A. K. Rush, (Random House)

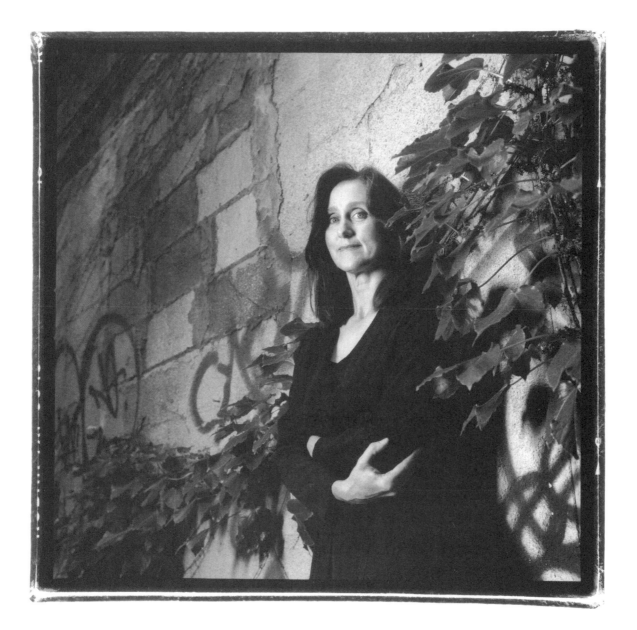

PATRICK HARBRON

Patrick Harbron has been photographing people for many years. His work has appeared in *Life, Time, Esquire, Los Angeles Times Magazine*, and others. He has received numerous awards for his portraits in magazines, books, annual reports, and advertising. Harbron lives in New York City with his wife, Dana.

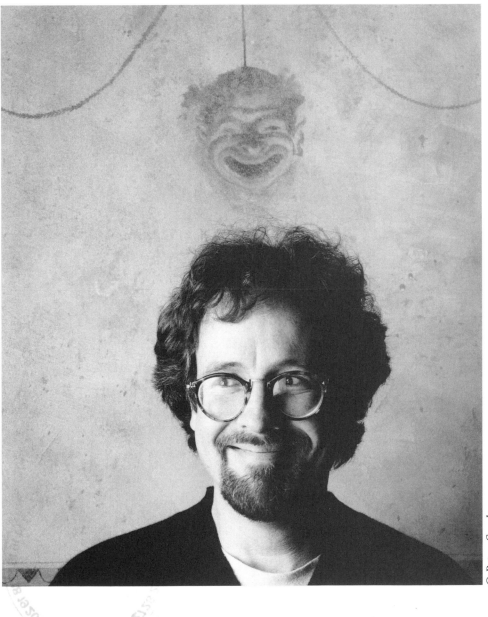

*Another day dawned all hot and fresh and, in persuance of
my unswerving policy at that time, I was singing "Sonny Boy"
in my bath, when Jeeves's voice filtered through the woodwork …
I had just got to that bit about the angels being lonely,
where you need every ounce of concentration in order to make
the spectacular finish, but I signed off courteously.*
—P.G. Wodehouse
"Jeeves and the Song of Songs"